Praise f(
The Sensc

"If you're the parent, teacher, relative or friend of a sensory kid, *The Sensory Processing Diet* will give you unique insight into his or her world. Chynna does an incredible job of taking a complex neurological condition and breaking it down in a way that is accessible and easy to understand. Based on her experience as a parent of a child with sensory needs, Chynna gives tangible and practical advice for mitigating the effects of sensory processing issues. Reading it was a breath of fresh air, as I could relate to so many of her parenting struggles and found her recommended interventions to be both doable and helpful. *The Sensory Processing Diet* is my new 'Bible' for all things sensory processing. Thank you, Chynna, for this amazing resource."

— CAMERON KLEIMO, sensory mom

"Chynna Laird has written a sensational book about a little known disorder, but one that is becoming increasingly more identified in children. She deconstructs the mystery of Sensory Processing Disorder and shares information from both a scientific and personal point of view. As a child psychologist, I found the book to be interesting, informative and complete. It offers a wide range of information and resources, as well as a level of detail that will be appreciated by the reader. I recommend it highly to parents and professionals. I loved it."
—LAURIE ZELINGER, PhD, ABPP, RPT-S, board certified psychologist, author of *Please Explain "Anxiety" to Me*

"I work with many children in play therapy that also experience sensory issues. This is a comprehensive and practical resource, both for parents and for those who help children experience sensory processing disorder (SPD). The author gives an in depth look at contributors to SPD, what types of treatments are available and adjustments families and children can make so that a child with SPD can cope in life in a way that he/she hasn't understood before. I whole heartedly recommend *The Sensory Processing Diet* to therapists and parents."
—JILL OSBORNE, EDS, LPC, CPCS, RPTS, author of *Sam Feels Better Now!*

The Sensory Processing Diet

One Mom's Path of Creating Brain, Body and Nutritional Health for Children with SPD

Chynna Laird

Loving Healing Press

Ann Arbor, MI

Library of Congress Cataloging-in-Publication Data

Names: Laird, Chynna T., 1970- author.
Title: The sensory processing diet : one mom's path of creating brain, body
    and nutritional health for children with SPD / Chynna Laird.
Description: Ann Arbor, MI : Loving Healing Press, [2020] | Includes
    bibliographical references and index. | Summary: "The Sensory Diet is
    not just about nutrition, it prescribes a complete program to address
    all of the needs of a child growing up with Sensory Processing Disorder
    (SPD) including exercises and evaluation methods for exteroceptors
    (visual, auditory, gustatory, olfactory, and tactile senses),
    proprioceptors (vestibular, proprioceptive) and interoceptors. The
    holistic approach is required because SPD can affect almost every aspect
    of the nervous system"-- Provided by publisher.
Identifiers: LCCN 2020027613 (print) | LCCN 2020027614 (ebook) | ISBN
    9781615995219 (trade paperback) | ISBN 9781615995226 (hardback) |
    ISBN
    9781615995233 (adobe pdf) | ISBN 9781615995233 (kindle edition)
Subjects: LCSH: Sensory integration dysfunction in children--Alternative
    treatment--Popular works. | Sensory disorders in
    children--Patients--Diet therapy--Popular works.
Classification: LCC RJ496.S44 L36 2020 (print) | LCC RJ496.S44 (ebook) |
    DDC 618.92/8--dc23
LC record available at https://lccn.loc.gov/2020027613
LC ebook record available at https://lccn.loc.gov/2020027614

Published by Loving Healing Press
5145 Pontiac Trail
Ann Arbor, MI 48105

www.LHPress.com
info@LHPress.com
Tollfree (USA/CAN/PR): 888-761-6268
FAX: 734-663-6861

Distributed by Ingram Group (USA/CAN/AU), Bertram Books (UK/EU),
New Leaf (USA)

Audiobook editions at Audible.com, iTunes, and Amazon

Contents

Foreword by Shane Steadman

It is estimated that one out of six children deal with some type of Sensory Processing Disorder (SPD). Yet, it is still one of the more unrecognized issues that plague our children as they try to function throughout their daily activities at home, school and with peers. Chynna Laird's book, *The Sensory Processing Diet: One Mom's Path of Creating Brain, Body and Nutritional Health for Children with SPD* presents a simplistic, informative and extremely useful guide for parents who are frustrated and struggle with the daily routines of their children with SPD. Unfortunately, these routines are met with sensory integration disturbances (feeding, behavior and playing with others). There is now a book from a parent to a parent.

I talk regularly with parents and work with kids who have some type of developmental delay. Besides developing nutritional and neurological treatment plans for these kids, my staff and I spend much of our time educating parents and providing resources that support them on the their difficult journey. Chynna Laird's book is a great resource and offers the tools necessary for parents to deal with the day-to-day struggle. When I read the book for the first time, I was impressed to see a list of what parents can do for their children at home as well as how to interact and engage their kids in a school setting. It was also exciting to see the many websites that parents can reference and get even more ideas that help. Equipping and empowering the parents is important in making any treatment plan successful.

Many parents who seek a diagnosis of their children often feel intimidated by the name of the condition. It almost seems like a sentencing of sorts. They often think to themselves, "Now what?" and go from practitioner to practitioner looking for some kind of answer to their diagnosis. Or, they search the Internet and are frightened by what they read. This book is very valuable, as it gives an overview of how the brain functions, therapies for the brain (the sensory diet), and resources for parents to gain more information.

The first section of the book gives a simplified and easy-to-understand description of how the brain works. I find that many people have no idea what really goes on inside our heads, and sometimes they are not sure if they want to find out. Chynna's explanations of how the brain communicates with the body through concepts like the 'VP of Operations', 'Departments' and 'Bicycle Messengers' help to make sense of what your child is experiencing.

The next section provides creative ideas for how to interact with and help your child who is suffering with SPD. It is amazing how much parents can do with and for their children. *At-Home Strategies for Managing Sensory Processing Disorder* is full of ideas for parents that are simple to use and provide great interaction with their children, thereby creating a bond. Once a parent gets the concepts of interacting while doing therapy, the possibilities become enormous. One of my favorite and easy-to-incorporate games from the book is called, 'Fun With Boxes'. Many kids like playing with boxes and for a parent to get inside a box and play with their kids is a great therapy tool as well as a great bonding experience.

Another section gives parents helpful hints when working with schools. Often parents comment on how hard it is to have a kid with SPD in school. I find that teachers are willing to help, but they often are unsure of what to do. By sharing ideas and ways to communicate with schools and different groups, this book can help relieve some of the frustration for parents, teachers and students.

At the end of the book, Chynna provides many websites and resources to help parents continue the learning process. These resources include educational material, recipes, websites and even ideas for toys. A great recipe in the book to try is the gluten-free chicken nuggets. Many parents think that getting their kids to eat something healthy is impossible. If you find recipes that taste great and make your kids feel like they're eating the same things as all of the other kids, it becomes easier than you might think.

I highly recommend this book both to parents who are just beginning their journey and to those who feel like they're on a never-ending treadmill. It is great to see a book written for the point of view of a parent who has gone through the struggles, since she can relate with what readers are going through. I hope that you enjoy the book as much as I did and use the many resources along your journey.

Shane Steadman, DC

Dr. Shane Steadman is one of a small handful of chiropractic neurologists in the state of Colorado and is an expert in peripheral neuropathy. He is a sought-after speaker and expert, regularly appearing in the media and is the co-owner of Mountain Health Chiropractic & Neurology Center, LLC.

Foreword by Kelly Dorfman, M.S., L.N.D.

As a nutritionist, I am very excited to be writing the Foreword to a book about Sensory Processing Disorder (SPD). Over the last 15 years, I have traveled around the country pounding the metaphoric drum about the connection between nutritional issues and SPD problems. In my experience, often the sensory system cannot be fixed without improving the nutritional environment in which it operates. Conversely, picky eaters can have sensory problems that need to be addressed before the diet will improve.

More than 20 years ago I started to see children who were developing normally and then suddenly stopped. One child was speaking two languages at his second birthday and a month later was non-verbal and diagnosed with autism spectrum disorder. At the time, autism was thought to be a condition a child was born with. There was no recognized diagnosis to explain regression at 18 months. Parents were told they had just *thought* the child was talking, or they were just dismissed as delusional about their offspring. How the world has changed!

My philosophy is that the parent is always right until proven otherwise. It was immensely disturbing to watch these parents suffer and have no ideas what to do. By the fourth case (in one month), I decided that I would either find answers or make them up!

Children who have sensory issues tend to be more vulnerable to having nutritional and/or digestive issues. If children start with sensory issues (as in premature infants, for example), their experiences are different from ours. The primitive nervous system needs to be fully operational for a child to read and interpret information accurately. What others see as pleasure, the child may experience as pain. When there is a lot of information, they may not know what to focus on.

Eating is such a sensory banquet. Everything you can think of that involves the sensory system is involved in the eating process: temperature, texture, taste, smell, sounds, color and/or pressure. It is one activity that involves every aspect of sensory input. So, if your reading and collating of sensory data is off, eating is almost always affected.

The vast majority of children with sensory issues are picky eaters. A small percentage of them are overeaters or indiscriminate eaters. So predominate are eating issues among children with Sensory Processing Disorder that if a parent tells me her child has no problems with food, I suspect the Sensory Processing Disorder (SPD) diagnosis is either wrong or I know the problem is mild.

Incorporating a nutritional overhaul can assist with easing a sensory-sensitive child's behavioral and emotional difficulties. How? The neurological therapy one does to correct SPD, such as occupational therapy (OT), needs a biochemical base to hold it. The sensory system is the nervous system. It is just that the parts, like the vestibular system, are embedded in the brain, so you don't see them like you see your ears. You can have corrective sensory treatment, but if the chemistry of the nervous system is not optimal, the body will not hold the corrections. It is like going to a chiropractor with a broken back and expecting exercises and adjustments to work.

Children behave in certain ways for a reason. We can blame the parents or label them as spoiled, but I think they are trying the best they can within the system they are operating. Look at what your picky eater is consuming. Imagine yourself eating that same meal plan (or snack plan in many cases). Most people have no trouble imagining how they would feel on a diet of bagels, crackers and macaroni and cheese. Lousy. Cranky. Volatile. Just like their kid feels.

A study by Brown & Matheny (1971) with twins found a measurable IQ difference when one twin was a picky eater and one ate a balanced diet. The picky eater, especially if he was a boy, performed more poorly on the IQ test. Many researchers like to use twins because the genetics and much of the rest of the environment is the same.

The authors said, "This study utilized such reported difference within young twin pairs to show that subtle variations in eating habits in the first year, an important period for brain growth and development, can be related to difference in mental abilities".

Sensory processing is a primitive mental function but critical for optimal cognitive and physical development. What is more surprising is that we expect youngsters' engines to run optimally on bad fuel. "Oh, they were just going through a phase," the worried parent is told. Or, "All kids eat like that." Some nutrients, such as fats, are structural. That means, you literally put them into your body as you would put a brick into a wall. The right fat creates one structure that has a certain kind of function while a different fat will build a different structure with altered function. In animal studies, when rats are given the kind of fats found in highly processed fast food and snacks, they could not learn how to run through mazes. In another study, they did not want to socialize with other rats when they were fed inferior diets.

The chemistry of the body matters. So a parent should take control of her "sensational" child's nutrition as soon as that little voice in her head that says, "Mayday!" starts talking. First, gather information, such as the type in this book. Next, close the gap between what the child is willing to eat and what they need for optimal brain development using nutritional supplements. You may need a professional to help you figure out what you need and how to get it in place. Third, get the help you need.

Being concerned for your child's welfare does not automatically brand you as an over-anxious parent. If you are concerned, there is likely an excellent reason. No, your child cannot thrive on a diet of three foods unless those three foods are chard, fish and brown rice. Even then, we would have to add some calcium, vitamin C and vitamin D.

When you add a sensory diet to your child's life, it rewires nervous system function. Every time you have an experience, there is a neurological action that goes with that experience. Let's say you are bouncing on a ball, for example. Your brain now has to process pressure information (from your backside). The part of your brain that reads proprioceptor information is now flooded with repetitive pressure information. The neurons there are firing over and over with every bounce.

Once those neurons are firing many, many times the brain has to make an adjustment. In the beginning, the neurons talk one to the next in a tentative way because they have never fired in that direction before. A neuron (nerve cell) in your brain can have anywhere between 10,000 and 100,000 connections when operating in a mature, complex brain. When one fires a group of neurons together over and over, the number of connections starts to increase so that it is easier to run that pathway. Your body reasons that you continue to do this activity, so it must be important. Chemical changes occur to make it easier to fire these neurons, and once one gets going, your body gets used to this activity so the whole group fires together more smoothly. This is the chemistry of learning.

Once the pathways get to a certain point of development, you need new information to build more complexity. In learning disabilities or

SPD, the child keeps having the experience, yet the learning does not occur or persist. The child can bounce for hours and never seem to get tired of it or turn the bouncing into the basis for new learning. ("We have bounced enough and know how to read pressure. Now let's try something imaginative like playing dress up".)

The right program for your child will involve a combination of the balanced chemistry (diet) and the specific evolving sensory activities that will help your child's brain so it can take in and process new information better. Do nutritional deficits cause sensory processing disorders? Yes. Do sensory processing disorders cause eating problems? Yes. Which comes first? Here is a classic chicken-or-egg dilemma that will keep cocktail party conversation going for hours. Chynna, along with many other parents, doctors and therapists, has recognized the important relationship between nutrition and the nervous system and the need to address one side to fix the other. This book will help you figure out what that might look like in your unique situation.

Kelly Dorfman, M.S., L.N.D.

Acknowledgments

I have so many people I'd like to thank for making this book what I hoped it would become. And I hope I remember every one.

First, I thank Dr. Lucy Miller for carrying on Dr. Ayres' work. Without you, there wouldn't be the fabulous OTs out there teaching our children how to live in our world with us the way they truly want to.

I am so grateful to Kathy Mulka and her wonderful team of occupational therapists who have not only worked miracles with my children, but who have also filled in the blanks with this often-confusing and overwhelming disorder so that I can be a better parent to my kids.

Thank you to Jen for sharing your personal success story. I love putting other caregivers in the spotlight, and you certainly deserve to be there. Thank you to Kelly Dorfman, Dana Laake, Dr. Shane Steadman, Krysten Hager and Jane Hersey for your expertise and sharing your wisdom and insight. I am so fortunate to know such incredible people.

Thank you to Victor Volkman, and all the folks at Loving, Healing Press for believing in me, my children and our projects on SPD. With his support, we have created different ways of helping these families learn to cope with this disorder in their own way. Special thanks to Laurie Zelinger, PhD, ABPP, RPT-S, a board certified psychologist who provided last minute technical and editorial assistance.

Last, but certainly not least, I am so, so grateful to my little family. "Mom" for being my #1 fan, Ryan for helping me out when deadlines needed to be met and to my four little babies. You all continue to inspire me each and every day with your beautiful faces, your belly laughs and your never-ending energy.

This book is a loving mixture of our own experiences with the information from the experts you should keep close at hand.

I hope with all of my heart, it helps you along your own 'sensational' journey. (When I say "sensational child", this is just shorthand for "a child with Sensory Processing Disorder (SPD)" in this book.)

Introduction

When my fifteen-year old daughter was diagnosed with Sensory Processing Disorder (SPD) 13 years ago, we were lost in terms of what to do for her. We'd lived with her 'quirks' (the name we gave to her severe behaviors and reactions to things) for so long and thought we'd been coping pretty well. What we didn't realize at the time was that our 'coping strategies' weren't really helping in the right way. In fact, we were unknowingly *adding* to her struggles.

Our house had become almost like a battleground with the enemy sneaking up on us at any moment of the day, silent and without warning. After a while, we learned what set off our daughter's melt-downs, and instead of facing hours of trying unsuccessfully to calm her *after* an event, visit, shopping trip or other experience, we timed such things to the second before the meltdown was eminent or simply avoided experiences completely.

My child's fear of the outside world became so intense, there were days I had to physically force her out on the front lawn just to get some fresh air and sunshine (in the most loving, supportive way I could, of course). And it grew to become complete isolation for our family.

In the earlier years, we did the best we could without knowing what our daughter was dealing with. But I also knew that how we were handling things wasn't helping. How could it? She wasn't experiencing her childhood the way she should have been, and it hurt me to watch her staring out our living room window watching other kids running and playing. But her sensitivity to things, mostly noise, smells and *especially* touch, were so severe that it literally took hours to bring her down from any sort of stimulation.

If it was too windy; if the lawn care guys were doing their job; if it was too sunny; if there were too many kids around her; if the lights in a store were 'flickery'; if someone dared to come over and say, "Hi!"; if her clothes didn't feel right, she cried, screamed and even clawed at her eyes, ears, or skin until we brought her back home to her 'safe place'. I knew I had to take more assertive steps in getting her what she needed.

The first professional who worked with our daughter, a loving occupational therapist (OT) named Donna Gravelle, said to me one day after our weekly at-home sessions, "You have to encourage this little girl to get out there and experience the world the best way she can. Otherwise she'll never learn that the world doesn't have to be such a scary place."

After two years of different sorts of therapy, with nothing working the way it should have, a psychiatrist 'strongly suggested' that we put our daughter on medication to ease her anxiety. Needless to say, we were shocked.

"Surely there have to be other ways to treat a three-year-old child than with drugs," I said in response. "There have to be other options, *better* options, for us to try before we'd even consider that."

That's actually a nicer way to describe what I'd said, but the point is that we wanted to treat our daughter holistically and without medication. That didn't mean we were 'anti-medication'. We were parents at the beginning of our journey with SPD and believed there must have been so many options available to try first.

The most important of the options that we discovered later was called the Sensory Diet. Note that the word *diet* here refers to a *regimen* or *program*. It is not specific to nutritional intake, although nutrition works very closely in the treatment process. And it was Donna who made it clear to us just how important the Sensory Diet is for a child with SPD.

At first, when Donna tried to explain to me how much my daughter needed a sensory diet, I have to admit I was a bit defensive. How could *she* know what my daughter needed? I had done everything I could to make the world safe for her. I knew exactly what things / people /experiences / clothes / etc. set her off, and I did everything in my power to make her feel better about those things / people / experiences / clothes / etc. even if I had to remove or avoid them. How *dare* Donna say that my child needed something else! But once I fully absorbed what she had said, I realized how right she was.

You see, by allowing my daughter to hide out in the sanctity of our home and helping her to avoid potentially sensory stimulating things, I was adding to her problem. I wasn't teaching her how to face things head-on. Instead, I helped her keep everything away that *might have had* a negative impact on her so that she didn't have to feel uncomfortable or scared. No wonder her reactions to things worsened over time.

She wasn't learning how to be in tune enough with her body to be able to say, "Okay, _____ makes me feel _____, so I have to _____ to feel better." *That's* how we help these children. By experiencing things in a fun, safe way so they learn how to function in the world around them. As Carol Stock Kranowitz (author of the book *The Out Of Sync Child*) has said time and time again, "Children learn when they're moving... and that's critical for children with dysfunction of sensory integration, or SPD.

I've learned two invaluable lessons in the past thirteen years of dealing with SPD in two of my four children. The first lesson was letting go of the belief that I could do it all by myself. My children needed a trained expert in SPD and sensory sensitivity to teach *all of us* how to help them. These children thrive best when everyone around them supports, nurtures and learns right beside them.

The second lesson was that knowledge is power. Believe me, if I'd known back then all that I know now, things may have been so different. But we can never look back. We can only look forward to brighter and better things. And that's what I hope to help you achieve with this book.

This book is all about the Sensory Diet---why we do it, what we need to make it work, who's involved and what should happen. Yes, there are many ups and downs and this book also delves into several of those other concerns, such as discipline, school and even other disorders that can be inter-related, or comorbid with SPD (e.g. ADHD, anxiety or OCD) and how the diet can also help in these areas.

It took me a long time to realize that in order to advocate for my children, I had to understand everything about their disorder, including all the best ways to help them. Once I reached that level of under-standing, I was finally able to help others understand SPD too. After all, if these children are learning how to cope in the world with others then we should be willing to do our part to help them achieve success.

From the bottom of my heart, and to all of those helping me bring this information to other parents, thank you.

<table>
<tr><td>

1

</td><td>

Your Child's Brain and Sensory Processing Disorder (SPD)

</td></tr>
</table>

If you are reading this book, it is likely that your child has recently been diagnosed with Sensory Processing Disorder (SPD). This is probably alarming and confusing. It may be the first time you've ever heard of this condition. What is it? How did my child get it? What can I do about it?

You may be unfamiliar with neurology lingo and have little use for highly technical explanations of SPD. However, in order to be of the best possible help to your child in navigating through the struggles ahead, it is very important that you gain a layman's understanding of what SPD is.

When I first heard about SPD, I was told that it was a disorder that interferes with how the brain communicates with the rest of the body. I wanted to understand this basic definition better, so I decided to learn as much as I could about the entire nervous system.

Arming yourself with the layman's version of the brain and nervous system gives you several advantages:

- Once you understand how a properly functioning system is supposed to work, you'll be able to see your child in an entirely new light. Most people can handle almost anything if they are armed with the right information. When my daughter was first diagnosed, I talked to therapists, psychologists and other parents. I also took courses on the brain and child development. Learning about the brain and its various functions is essential because in doing so you will better understand SPD and what you're dealing with. You'll find answers to all of those 'what' questions. But learning about the brain and nervous system answers the 'why' questions, such as, "Why does this sensation bother her so much when another one doesn't?" or "Why can't she run, jump and stay balanced?" and "Why can she create gorgeous pictures, but is not able to hold a pencil to write properly or coordinate her hands to use scissors?" Having that knowledge can be both comforting and empowering.

- Knowing more about the brain and nervous system helps you step back and identify possible causes of the behaviors you're seeing in your child. Understanding what the triggers are enables you to help your child manage his behaviors more effectively.

- SPD has often been termed as an 'invisible' disorder because you can't see it on a child's face or body and you can't give a child pills to make it go away. Absorbing as much information as we can empowers us to be strong advocates for our children, because we know that they don't simply have behavioral problems, but are actually struggling with something much deeper.

- The more we understand about the disorder, and the systems and organs it affects, the better we can help educate others. After all, our children are learning how to function in the world around them and with the people in it. Shouldn't those same people understand how to interact with our children too? Unfortunately, caregivers and educators who don't know about SPD, or understand how it truly affects the body, may punish the child for her overt behavior instead of digging for the root of the reactions.

The Nervous System – Our Body's Messenger System

I was taught to think of the nervous system as a huge messaging corporation made up of the Head Office (the brain, pun intended), the central messaging track (spinal cord) and the micro-messaging routes (peripheral system). And, of course, there are the little bicycle messengers and messenger assistants (the neurons and neurotransmitters) that take the brain's messages everywhere they're supposed to go.

I will briefly go over these different areas in order to understand how the whole system works together, and then discuss how SPD interferes with the nervous system's ability to do its job effectively.

The Head Office: the Brain

Considering its size, only about 2.9 pounds (or 1.3 kilograms), it is amazing how many tiny structures there are inside the human brain and how all of those tiny structures work together taking in, processing and sending out information to help our bodies function most effectively. And because of this need for unity, dysfunction in one area of the brain can impact functioning in other areas, which can result in the body not getting clear messages about what it's supposed to be doing. A lot of SPD research focuses on the areas and structures in the brain relating to sensation, emotion, motivated behavior, movement, attention, sleep and maintenance of muscle tone.

The head office of our messaging corporation is divided into two departments (*hemispheres*), which communicate the 'goings-on' of the rest of the corporation through a thin, but strong, wall (*corpus callosum*). Now each of these main departments has its own special jobs and functions (*lateralization*), but they work as a team to get other members of the corporation to do their jobs efficiently and properly.

The head office divvies up jobs fairly by dividing the main departments into mini areas (*lobes*) that are each in charge of specific bodily functions:

- *Frontal* deals with behavior, personality, control of movement and learning.

- *Parietal* mostly helps out with *proprioception* (perception or awareness of the position and movement of the body) as well as processing tactile and visual information

- *Temporal* takes on tasks having to do with coordinating hearing and speech and,

- *Occipital* in the back of the brain, deals with vision and helping the brain to understand what the eyes are seeing.

Before messages get to the head office, the VP of Operations (*brain stem*) stops them and decides which area of the head office each message should go to for processing and suggests an appropriate course of action. The VP has assistants to read messages about balance, equilibrium and coordination (*cerebellum*) and helps determine the meaning of those messages (*limbic system*). From there, messages are then analyzed by the VP of Central Processing (*cerebral cortex*) before being sent back into the messaging system, since it has final say on the processing of sensory and motor information for the corporate body.

Once this procedure is complete, which actually takes mere seconds, the response is shipped out of the VP of Operations area to the messaging track (*spinal cord*) to reach its final destination.

Although this is an extremely simplified explanation, it really is all a parent needs to know at this point. The most important thing to remember is that the connection of these messages is very important because if they get mixed up, or stopped, at any other point, the receiver won't know what's going on.

According to Dr. A. Jean Ayres, who was a Masters-level occupational therapist, a Ph.D. in educational psychology and credited for discovering SPD, the areas in the brain specialized to one sense receive information and respond simultaneously to more than one sort of sensation at a time.

Here's an example of how sensory and motor senses work together. If you gave a baby a rattle, it could be a brightly colored or shiny silver one that feels cold/smooth/textured in some way and makes noise when shaken. The sensory systems involved with vision, tactile, hearing, fine motor skills (to grasp the rattle), and coordination will have to work together to give the child the information he or she needs to interact properly with the rattle. So, you see how things can be a little confusing, even for something as basic as playing with a toy, when messages aren't being processed properly.

The Spinal Cord: The Message Track

Essentially, the spinal cord's job is to carry sensory and motor input messages to the brain, as well as response messages from the brain to the rest of the body. Using our messaging system analogy, messages travel along the messaging track to the head office for processing, then the responses are brought back to their final destination in the corporate body for action.

There really isn't much sensory processing going on in the spinal cord, but it's important to understand what's happening in there because some of the exercises in later chapters involved stimulating and stretching out the spinal cord to help it do its job more effectively.

Neurons and Neurotransmitters: The Transporters and Bicycle Messengers

Neurons are defined as brain cells that send and receive messages using electrical impulses. *Neurotransmitters* are the chemicals that help the neurons communicate with one another. So going back to our messenger model, messages are taken from the messaging track (*spinal cord*) by the bicycle messengers (*neurons*), who transport the important messages to a small sorting area (*synapse*) that stop the message in order to decide what the next bicycle messenger should do with it. Once a decision is made, the messenger assistants send the message along on its journey. The message actually makes several stops like this along its way before it reaches its final destination. It is like a relay race in which one runner goes a certain distance, then passes the baton to the next runner waiting.

As long as the messenger assistants interpret the messages correctly, or don't lose them somehow, it's usually a smooth run.

The Peripheral Nervous System (PNS): The Body's Micro-Messaging Routes

This division of our message corporation is where messages travel on their journey after processing, or on their way up for processing. It's the route the bicycle messengers follow. It sort of resembles a spider web stemming from the spinal cord out to the rest of the body. SPD researchers are interested in this area because it is in charge of delivering the messages that instruct the body how to react to, or even *whether* to react to, sensory stimulation.

The micro-messaging route (*PNS*) is sub-divided into two main parts:

- **The somatic nervous system,** which is the section that helps us interact with our environments. It contains sensory bicycle messengers (*afferent nerves*) that carry the sensory message from skin, skeletal muscle, joints, eyes, ears, etc. to the nervous system and motor bicycle guys (*efferent nerves*), which carry motor messages from the brain and spine to the skeletal muscles.

- **The autonomic or sensory nervous system,** which is in charge of the functions in our bodies that we aren't consciously aware of. This system also has afferent nerves that carry sensory messages from the organs to the brain and efferent nerves that carry motor messages from the brain to the internal organs. This system has smaller sub-divisions called the *parasympathetic nervous system* and the *sympathetic nervous system*. These systems are discussed in greater detail in Chapter 2, which discusses the interoceptors. For now, all you need to remember is that the sympathetic system prepares us to deal with stress or danger – the heartbeat increases, our breathing rate increases, we become more aware of sensory stimulation – due to an increase of adrenaline in the system. The parasympathetic system, on the other hand, is what's in charge of bringing the body back down and keeping it in a homeostatic, or calm, state.

Why do you need to know all of this? Because neurons and brain structures can be working perfectly fine, but the neurotransmitters that help carry the message to the next neuron in line may not know how to interpret that message. This results in the final message being misinterpreted or scrambled, resulting in the brain and body not understanding what to do. It's sort of like play the game 'telephone' where a group of people are in a line and the first person whispers something to the person next to him. That person then whispers the message they heard to the next person and the message gets repeated in a whisper from one person to the next down the line until the last person says aloud what she heard. Often the final message isn't even close to what the original person had said.

As you'll find out in Chapter 3, the Sensory Diet is how we help our children 'unscramble' those messages so they're able to function better.

In summary, your child with SPD doesn't have a *brain* problem. He has a *connection* problem. But with the right mixture of nutrition, exercises and other sensory activities, your child's connections can be helped along to do their job much more effectively.

And that's the whole focus of this book.

Why Can't We See SPD on an Ultrasound?

Why Is There No Blood Test to Confirm SPD?

SPD: An Invisible Disorder

These are two very common questions parents ask when their child is first diagnosed with SPD, and they are logical ones. After our children have gone through a rigorous assessment process in order to confirm sensory issues, as well as the severity level, there is still no one who can give us a solid, conclusive reason why our child has this disorder. This knowledge is important to parents. We need those answers so we can understand and face the diagnosis. The good news is that as time goes on, and more parents share their pearls of wisdom, that knowledge is spreading. And we are closer than ever to learning the answers we so desperately want to our many 'why' questions.

SPD has often been called an invisible disorder because you can't see it. There's nothing on the outside of these children to indicate they have something wrong with them other than their reactions to stimuli and their overt behavior. And that can be so frustrating when trying to take that first step in seeking help.

I wondered why, despite all the ultrasounds I'd had when I was pregnant, no one was able to see anything wrong with my daughter's brain. What I didn't realize then was that those technicians were only measuring the size of her brain and marking the development of the brain structures. They couldn't see SPD or monitor how it affected the brain structures because it's not like a tumor or other physical defect. It's invisible. A blood test wouldn't tell you whether SPD is present either because it isn't in the bloodstream. It's deep in the circuitry of the nervous system.

As mentioned earlier in this chapter, SPD is considered a *connection* problem. We can't see that those messages aren't getting through or that the brain struggles to read them. In utero, the brain is still developing and as long as the technicians can see limbs moving and the heart beating, they assume the brain is doing its initial job. There are no visible indications of SPD until the baby comes into the world and tries interacting with their environment.

How Does SPD Interfere With the Brain's Job?

Now that you have a basic understanding of how the brain, nervous system and sensory systems work together as a team to help process sensory information effectively, it's equally as important to also have a solid understanding of what happens to that well-functioning system when a child has SPD.

I've come to learn that there's a huge difference between *knowing about* something and *understanding* it. It's vital that parents understand exactly what SPD is, what it isn't and why the Sensory Diet is essential in helping their children function in, and interact effectively with, the world around them. Plus, understanding this disorder empowers parents to be the strongest advocates they can be for their child.

When my daughter was diagnosed with SPD, I was relieved to finally understand what she'd been struggling with, but I also felt lost and powerless at the same time. Not only did I still not understand what was wrong with her most of the time (even *after* the diagnosis), but I also never knew the right way to help her. And often the things I tried only made her reactions worse. As I figured out later on, I wasn't doing the *right* activities at the *right* times, so my attempts to help her were more irritating for her than soothing.

On top of that, raw feelings of immense guilt for not being able comfort my own child were intensified when I was told I needed extra help in caring for her. That was hurtful and hard to accept at first, but I knew I had to do something. She'd suffered so much already to that point and was literally trapped inside of herself. She needed someone to free her, and I needed someone to help me learn how to maintain that freedom.

In retrospect, I realize there's nothing wrong with accepting outside help. There's truth to the old expression, "It takes a village to raise a child". It doesn't mean others have to take care of a child because the parents *can't*. It means that there are people out there who are experts in certain areas who can help fill in the gaps within our own parental expertise. And so, with the help of a loving, caring and knowledgeable occupational therapist (OT), I learned how to pay closer attention to my child's reactions in various situations, was coached on figuring out her triggers and was taught how to identify which parts of her Sensory Diet she needed and when.

The following sections help to make aspects of the disorder clear so parents and caregivers understand what their child's diet is supposed to do and recognize signs when more intense treatment options may be required. You may already be well-informed on the details of this chapter, but it's always handy to have extra information on SPD to refer to for the later chapters on specific methods for each sensory system.

Understanding Dysfunction in Sensory Integration

Earlier in this chapter I discussed the parts of the brain and nervous system and how a properly functioning system works. Understanding, generally, how this system works and how it's supposed to respond to sensory stimulation can help you understand how SPD interferes with this functioning.

The first thing to grasp is the concept of sensory integration. A word parents will hear a lot during their child's treatment sessions is *organization*. Helping to organize the child's body to cope with the world around him or her is the main goal in any sort of sensory integration therapy.

Here's one way to look at it. Most of us don't even think about every little sound, smell or other stimulus around us. Our sensory organs take information in and send it to the brain, which then analyzes the messages, sorts them and sends them on to the rest of the body to react (or not react) to. Essentially then, sensory integration is the brain's ability to organize and process the sensory messages it receives from the environment.

For a person with a dysfunction in this ability, the messages get misinterpreted somewhere along their journey, causing a backlog of information. The brain can't read these messages, so it can neither process them nor let the rest of the body know how to react to the sensations it experiences. This can cause a lot of problems.

Without this organizational ability, the body isn't able to interact with the environment the way it should. If messages aren't being processed properly, your child has difficulty learning the difference between good or bad sensations, how her body is supposed to move in space, or how he is supposed to react to certain people, objects or experiences. She may have trouble focusing on a task at hand because her brain isn't able to tell her what she needs to pay attention to and what she can ignore. And she may even have trouble with coordination, walking, or simple tasks such as using a pencil, cutting with scissors or playing with toys. This is because her body isn't getting the messages to move the way it should. Being that disorganized can be a scary, isolating experience, especially for a child. And it can also be dangerous.

My daughter always avoided sensory stimulation. Her senses were heightened all of the time, so even the slightest touch or sound was enough to send her into overdrive. But occasionally, she was completely the opposite. For example, when she was about two, I turned around for a moment to grab the shampoo and a few of her bathtub toys. In those few seconds, she'd reached up and turned on the water. What was odd was that she never flinched when the water sprayed all over her torso. In fact, I thought that she'd turned the cold tap on. That would have explained the initial lack of reaction since I'd just turned the taps off and the cold tap would have still have been running warmer until it cooled off again. But when I saw the steam rising from the water stream, I sprinted to shut the tap off. Her torso was deep red, and it took several more minutes before she reacted to the event. If I hadn't been right there, she would have scalded herself.

From this scenario, you can see how important it is to understand what goes on in a child's little body and the importance of helping him or her learn to organize themselves in preparation for our very sensory-rich world.

Opening the World's Eyes

Dr. A. Jean Ayres would be so proud of how far SPD research has come in unveiling this invisible disorder. In the late1960s and early '70s when she began her research, the technology available to researchers today simply didn't exist. Much of her research was observational at first, which is one reason why many people in the medical community don't agree with her findings. However, Dr. Ayres was a knowledgeable occupational therapist with experience and knowledge in neuroscience. She knew what to look for and what reactions/responses were connected to which areas of the brain. And her later research incorporated this in experiments with children who had sensory issues.

Today, fantastic researchers like Drs. Lucy Jane Miller and Jane Koomar have built upon Dr. Ayres's early research and have made phenomenal progress with the use of EEGs, MRIs and other accepted technological tools. Researchers are very close to finding the answers that parents and therapists need to better help our children.

What Causes SPD?

I asked our initial occupational therapist (OT) this very question because the books I'd read hadn't been very clear. Unfortunately, her answer was just as unclear. She said there could be many possible explanations for it, but nobody has been able to pinpoint it for certain. Currently, the most plausible explanations are genetic or hereditary predispositions, prenatal circumstances or birth trauma. But these are only *possible* explanations and not definite.

Researchers have discovered that the increase of environmental toxins in our world today (e.g.: pollution, viruses, teratogens, household cleaning products, hormones or additives in our food, etc.) that we breathe in, consume or otherwise come into contact with may contribute to dysfunction in sensory integration. This, combined with genetic considerations, such as the mother's physical, mental and neurological family history, can greatly contribute to the possibility of a child's vulnerability in developing SPD.

Some researchers believe that we women are incredibly likely to pass on the effects of toxins floating around in the environment to our children because after we ingest or take in these toxins, they are absorbed into our eggs. Our future babies! And we have no way of knowing if, or when, such damage has been done.

Dr. Ayres argued that genetic factors *can* make the brain in some children more vulnerable than usual to these environmental toxins. Brain development in utero is crucial to its future function and although, structurally, the child's brain may appear 'normal', the circuitry that helps run it may not be. Unfortunately, as stated earlier, these are not things that can be detected in an ultrasound. (See Suggested Reading and Resources to find more information on this subject.)

Babies' brains are also incredibly vulnerable during birth. If a baby is deprived of oxygen for a long period of time during or after birth, or if he experiences other sorts of birth trauma (e.g.: irregular or stopping of heartbeat, a very long labor, assisted birth methods, etc.), the brain's normal functioning and/or development may be affected.

Another possible cause of SPD often suggested by experts is the lack of a stimulating, sensory-rich environment. A child who has little contact with other people or objects can't develop properly functioning sensory, motor or intellectual functions. An example would be children in orphanages in underdeveloped countries or in other completely destitute places.

But it's not only children who are trapped in such extreme conditions that can be deprived of adequate sensory experiences. "Some parents don't know how to offer their child a completely satisfying sensory environment. One that meets the individual needs of the child," our occupational therapist (OT) explained to me once.

These parents aren't neglecting their children. They just don't know how to tell what kinds of sensory experiences their children needs. As a result, their children aren't interacting effectively with the toys or objects provided to them.

"We're here to help parents learn to pick up on what their child needs," said our OT of herself and other OTs' roles. "Then they can teach the child how to interact with the objects through play methods to give him the sensory input his body needs."

I was a bit defensive when I heard that. I mean, I provided my daughter with all sorts of things—music, touchy/feely books and toys and colorful baby objects. But, oddly enough, those were the very sorts of things, with the exception of music, that she was bothered by the most. Our OT wasn't suggesting that I wasn't parenting my child 'correctly', only that I needed to give her different sorts of stimulation in different ways so she could learn to experience them without fear.

The most interesting piece of information I learned was that once some parents learn what's wrong with their children, they actually say they remember experiencing similar feelings as children themselves. So, perhaps there *is* a genetic component causing the child to be predisposed to develop the disorder, but an environmental factor must also occur in order for SPD to surface.

Is SPD A 'Real' Diagnosis?

Parents whose children are diagnosed with SPD may ask themselves this initially. When my daughter received her diagnosis over thirteen years ago, I'd never heard of it. I'd heard of autism spectrum disorder (ASD) and attention deficit hyperactivity disorder (ADHD), but not this mysterious SPD. In fact, I had been taking a university brain and behavior course and my professor, Dr. John Piel, a well-known and highly respected Canadian neurologist, hadn't heard of it either. He told me that he actually had to Google SPD just to find out what I was asking him about. That both scared and angered me.

You see, although SPD was discovered in the late 1960s / early 1970s and has been researched for more than 35 years, there hasn't been enough massive, controlled, 'quantified' research to prove/disprove or predict symptoms or life course of the disorder. That's the pulse of research—to create a theory that survives as other researchers try to prove or disprove it. Because SPD has many symptoms that mimic other disorders, such as autism spectrum disorder and ADHD, to name only a couple, it is even more difficult to create a solid, controlled research environment.

Neurologists, such as Dr. Piel, don't typically consider SPD when testing and diagnosing children with sensory-related symptoms because their focus is on brain structures and developmental problems. A child with SPD cannot be given a blood test or MRI to 'see' the problem. Having said that, Dr. Lucy Miller's research team (through the STAR Institute) has taken pictures of a child's brain as well as noted physical reactions while experiencing specific sensory stimulation, but the child's physical reactions are not in sync. It's promising to see how close they are coming to identifying cause and effect.

According to www.sensory-processing-disorder.com (a prominent SPD website), other reasons for the difficulties encountered in researching SPD is that a child's symptoms can fluctuate from one day to the next, and even from one hour to another on some days. This makes it very difficult to find a controlled environment to conduct studies in, and the fluctuation in symptoms also makes it hard to find solid numbers to create statistics.

Additionally, SPD is considered a relatively new diagnosis, so there are many people who have it, even as adults, and don't even realize it. In fact, an example is a friend of mine who says she never knew why. She said her environment was sometimes a very uncomfortable and scary place for her while she was growing up. Imagine her surprise to be diagnosed at *age 35* with SPD. Then everything she'd gone through finally made sense to her.

All parents need to know is that today there is a much bigger pool of information and resources available at their fingertips to help their children learn to be all they can be without fear or question. You *can* make a difference. Don't give up.

The Sensory Systems: Exteroceptors, Proprioceptors and Interoceptors

What exactly does it mean when SPD experts tell you that your child's sensory systems are 'disorganized'? This chapter discusses each sensory system, the sensory receptors within each system, how the systems work when they are running properly and how SPD interferes with each system.

The Three Basic Parts of the Sensory System

The sensations we experience are often referred to as 'food' for the nervous system because without the right sensory nourishment, the nervous systems can't develop properly. The main sensory systems are grouped under three general categories:

- *Exteroceptors* include the most commonly understood sensory systems: visual (vision), auditory (hearing), olfactory (smell) and gustatory (taste). Also included in this category is tactile (touch). These five sense together are known as the Primary Systems because they give us the main information about our external environments and how we are supposed to relate to people and objects in that environment.

- *Proprioceptors* include the proprioceptive and vestibular sensory systems. These refer to how our bodies interact with our environments through balance, coordination, movement, gravity and our position in space. These systems are in charge of telling our bodies how to move and coordinate in the world, give us information about what our muscles and joints are doing and involve all aspects of fine and gross motor skills, from holding a pen, pencil or eating utensil, to bouncing a ball or jumping.

This chapter explains the basics about how each system is supposed to operate. The discussions of each system include short lists of general characteristics to refer to. This will help you to decide which exercises from the next few chapters your child needs the most and at which times of the day.

Exteroceptors: How Does the World Feel?

The Mozart concerto playing in the background, the luscious spices in the apple pie bubbling away in the oven or the light breeze blowing on your skin all send messages to your brain, which, in turn, then tells your body how to react to those sensations. Is it pleasant? Scary? Painful? Noisy? Rough? Stinky? Not being able to distinguish among these things can make coping in a sensory-rich world rather frightening at times.

In the beginning stages of our therapy and treatment process, our phenomenal OT gave me a wealth of information on the specific system she'd be working on with our daughter each week. This allowed me to not only understand what direction the OT was going in during therapy, but also what part of my child's brain she was attempting to organize. I found grasping this concept so important because when that therapist isn't there, we must rely on our own instincts.

The exteroceptors allow us to directly experience our world. And, as you'll discover, they work *together* to provide us with a complete sensory experience.

Sight (Visual)

Our sense of sight not only lets us see objects in our environment, but also helps us determine *how* we see those objects. Our sight also enables us to judge distance between objects, or between ourselves and objects, as well as how to move our bodies in relation to objects in our environment. Together, this is known as *visual perception*.

This system is amazing for several reasons. First, it almost entirely depends on light. Light waves bounce off of objects in various amounts, and then enter the eye. Second, the *optic nerve*, which is actually a whole bunch of those messenger routes bunched together, is directly connected to the visual cortices in the brain located just below the cerebellum. (If you remember our discussion of the brain, this part of the brain stem assists with interpreting the emotional response to stimuli in our environments.) Finally, the pathways in our visual system communicate directly with the spatial and motor areas that control eye and hand movement and spatial attention, as well as the recognition, identification and categorization of visual stimuli.

What all of this means is that people with SPD may:

- Not be able to determine how near to or far away from people, objects or other things they are.

- Have difficulty focusing on certain patterns or colors. (My kids, for example, always felt 'dizzy' when looking at zigzag patterns, spirals or stripes and didn't like looking at bright colors.)

- Feel fearful watching certain people's faces move when they're speaking.

- Bump into walls, furniture or people because they cannot judge how close they are or aren't able to see them properly.

- Say that sunlight or fluorescent light 'hurts' their eyes because the muscles in the eyes aren't coordinating with the receptors (*rods*, which help us see in low light and *cones*, which help us interpret color and work best in brighter light) in order to control the amount of light getting into the eye. (Both of my kids always needed sunglasses outside, as well as when we were in certain stores or certain people's houses.)

- Have difficulty following the words in books or under-standing visual forms of learning because they aren't able to focus their eyes properly.

- Not be able to see objects or people on one side of them or the other because the eyes aren't working *together* to give the brain that information.

- Not be able to 'tune out' action around them, distracting them from tasks at hand, because the brain can't tell them what they're supposed to be focusing on.

- Have difficulty with fine motor skills because the brain isn't able to properly coordinate eye and hand movements.

What set alarm bells off for me was that my daughter covered her eyes and screamed whenever we'd go outside or to the grocery store. Now, a lot of children react to having the sun blasting in their eyes when you're driving around in the car. But my kids, especially my daughter, reacted the same way in *any* sort of light as if it caused her great pain. Being cranky because the light is in the eyes is one thing. If that crankiness interferes with the child being able to play or relate to others or even results in him refusing to go outside or into certain places because 'it hurts', it is a sign that something else is going on.

Difficulty with vision can also interfere with a child's balance, how she interacts with people (e.g.: avoiding eye contact, what she'll play with, what looks good enough to eat or wear or even where she'll go). My daughter became so visually avoidant that any toys that were patterned, too bright, sprung out or moved too fast got tossed into her closet. She wouldn't wear clothes that were striped, heavily patterned or too bright. If her food didn't 'look right', and that didn't just mean texture-wise because it had a lot to do with color, she refused to eat. And if the lights in a store or a person's home were too bright or too dim, she didn't want to stay.

As a final point of interest, the optic nerves from each eye cross over at the base of the brain (*optic chiasm*) where the visual cortex is located. Because of this, information from the left eye gets sent for processing in the right side of the brain and vice versa. Knowing this may help parents understand that if messages aren't getting to where they're supposed to, their child may seem like they can't see objects on one side or the other, or why he may be looking right at something but not 'see' it. If the messages are getting stopped or blocked somewhere along their journey, the eyes can't work together and the child won't be able to see things properly or even get his hands to interact with an object the way he wants them to.

Hearing (Auditory)

Our sense of hearing relies on vibrations that are triggered by sounds waves. Different sounds in our environment create sound waves at different levels of frequency, which our brains help us to interpret as loud, soft, squeaky, gravelly or glass-shattering. The lower the pitch, the slower the vibration and the higher the pitch the faster it is. The receptors in the ear send auditory sensations to the *temporal lobe* for processing. Not only does the brain give us information about *what* we're hearing, it also tells us how to emotionally respond to auditory stimuli.

Think about a song that you love, the sound of fingernails scraping down a chalkboard or a baby crying. All of those sounds trigger different emotional responses in you, depending on how your brain interprets the information.

Hearing is closely related to language development. This is why children who have language or speech delays are sent for hearing tests to eliminate the possibility of hearing loss or some other underlying condition. If a child's brain isn't receiving sound stimuli from her environment, or the information simply isn't being processed properly, that child may not develop language and speech the same way other children do, if at all. Of course, hearing problems aren't the only possible cause of a child's language or speech struggles, but the two are often connected.

Finally, the receptors in the inner ear also impact aspects of the vestibular system such as balance, equilibrium and coordination. Have you ever been to a very loud concert and left the venue with ringing in your ears and feeling dizzy? Have you been held or hung upside down and felt that 'cotton in the ears' sensation? And if you've ever had an inner ear infection, you've most likely experienced the same sensations.

The reason for this is that one of the main parts of the auditory system, called the *cochlea* (which is swirl-shaped like a snail's shell), works directly with the vestibular system in sending and receiving sensory and motor information about where we are in relation to the world around us and in keeping us upright and moving.

Children with SPD may:

- Be frightened of loud or sudden noises, including certain pitched voices, thunder, sirens, vacuum cleaners or car horns.

- Become distressed from high-pitched sounds like whistles, screaming, baby cries, higher-pitch speaking or singing voices or squealing tires.

- Hear or notice sounds that most of us ignore, like toilets flushing, zippers or diaper tabs, Velcro or the humming sound some lights make.

- Have difficulty distinguishing between various noises presented together, such as when an orchestra plays or when there's a lot of noise in a room.

- Be unable to distinguish difference between tones, like whether a voice sounds mad or happy.

- Be unable to focus when someone is speaking to them or when doing an activity because of other noises around them.

- Have difficulty following lessons, discussions or conversations.

- Have difficulty keeping time with music or other music/ movement activities or recognizing /following rhymes. (This is known as *timbre*, which is being able to distinguish among different sounds.)

- Have difficulty distinguishing between words that sound similar.

- Have a shorter attention span and misunderstand questions.

- Need more repetition for directions or descriptions than usual.

- Have trouble with expressive language because their auditory systems aren't helping them learn how to speak, interact verbally or otherwise put their thoughts into words. Other signs include delay in speaking, a weak vocabulary, poor grammar, limited imaginative play and difficulty reading / following stories. My son struggled in all of these areas and not only needed to learn how to speak, but also be able to train his auditory receptors to understand what was being said to *him* so that he could respond.

- Struggle with speech in areas such as clarity, tone (e.g.: speaking too loudly or softly), or be hesitant about speaking at all.

The processing centers in the brain for visual and auditory information are located very close together and often exchange information. This could be why watching a movie with a beautiful soundtrack can impact us so strongly on an emotional level. It can also explain why children with sensory sensitivities are easily distracted and can experience sensory overload in busy, loud places.

Tasting (Gustatory) and Smelling (Olfactory)

Tasting and smelling are separate senses, but they influence each other so much that it makes sense to discuss them together. Think of what it's like when you have a cold and a stuffy nose. Can you taste anything? Not usually. Or think of moms out there who have such super-sensitive noses during pregnancy that smells can actually bring on nausea or vomiting? What we smell even effects what we're willing to taste.

If you look at your tongue in the mirror you can see tiny bumps called *taste buds*, which are the tongues sensory receptors. Those little buds help us to develop a good relationship with food. They give us four different taste sensations: sweet, sour, bitter and salty. Spicy is another taste sensation, but it is not usually categorized with the other four. These tastes are helpful in keeping harmful things out of our mouths and bodies because if something rancid or non-edible hits the tongue, it sends alarm signals to the brain to get rid of it. This is an essential survival instinct we're born with.

The olfactory system has sensory receptors in the nose. This system is unique in two ways. First, its sensory receptors depend on, and respond to, the chemical makeup of things in the environment that produce odors. And second, the system sends and receives messages about these smells right from the limbic system, bypassing the brain stem. This means that there is usually a direct and instant emotional connection to odors and scents that influences us to decide whether or not we like something or someone. Our olfactory system also creates strong memories that influence what products we buy and use and even what foods we eat.

The connection between these two systems, then, is that smell influences what we taste and even *how* we taste it. Together these systems create strong emotional memories for certain things, people, situations and events and these memories influence what we choose to surround ourselves with.

Knowing all of this can help you understand why your child may not want to be in certain stores or in people's homes. Or why she reacts adversely when you cook certain foods or put those foods on her plate. Or why being close to Daddy may bother her but being near Mommy doesn't.

When my daughter was very young, she fussed a lot more when her father held her than when I did. In normal cases, babies often prefer mom because they are usually with her more often and they may associate her scent with comfort, feeding and calmness. But it's not 'normal' for a child to refuse the same things from the other parent, or another person, simply because of their scent.

As my daughter got older, she related what she smelled to what we ate and, literally, stopped eating anything that wasn't plain. She avoided anything strong in flavor (such as spicier foods, garlic, most vegetables or sour fruits) or textured. The other concern, of course, is that if a child isn't eating well he won't be eliminating properly either, and that can be uncomfortable and even painful.

Children with SPD who struggle with gustatory and/or olfactory systems may:

- Display adverse reactions to strong smells or tastes.

- Alternatively, crave strong smells or tastes. My kids craved salty and sweet, which I curbed with healthier food choices. On bad days, when they weren't getting those cravings met, they'd stick non-edible items in their mouths to feel satisfied.

- Chew on or eat non-edible food items such as pencils, clothing, paintbrushes, paper, erasers or stuffed animals.

- Smell objects, toys or people.

- Gag around certain odors or even just thinking about those odors.

Another thing to keep in mind is that children with struggles in the olfactory/gustatory senses may also have what OTs call, 'oral motor problems'. This means that the muscles in and around the mouth and jaw, remembering that the tongue is a muscle, aren't getting proper messages about how to interact with food or other objects.

Other things to watch for are excessive drooling, speech delays, sucking on fingers or needing a pacifier more strongly than other children do. I discuss fine motor skills (eating and speaking are fine motor skills too) later in this chapter.

Tactile (Touching)

This is the sense of touch. The skin is the largest organ in the body. It covers us from head to toe, so we are constantly experiencing our world through our skin. It's been said that touch is the first sensation that develops *in utero* and helps babies experience their world while visual and other systems are still developing. It is also the most difficult to organize. We need the sense of touch to help our bodies feel organized and safe. In addition to feeling things, touching and being touched, this system also sends the brain messages about things like pressure on the skin, pressure, temperature, texture, pain and awareness of our bodies. When this system is out of whack, we don't feel safe in the world around us because we never know how something is going to feel.

Some children, for example, are intensely bothered by light touch. My daughter was, and it drove her crazy. When she was hyper-sensitive, she fought having a bath, getting her hair brushed or having her teeth brushed. She didn't like the feel of her clothes, wouldn't go outside if it was too windy or even refused to have anyone sit too close to her. To her, such things sent a 'pain' message to her brain and she went into immediate sensory overload.

There were other times, however, when she was able to shove her hands into snow, hold ice cubes, hit parts of her body on object or other people or touch something burning hot and she wouldn't feel the sensation until much later. This aspect of SPD, being under-responsive, is scarier because children can seriously injure themselves if they aren't able to respond to things quickly and effectively.

Tactile defensiveness or other struggles with touch are usually the first ones that become obvious to parents, so several of the following characteristics may already be familiar.

Your child may:

- Avoid being touched, including shying away from physical affection, such as hugging, kissing, cuddling, etc.

- Turn his head when being touched on the face or near it.

- Display abnormal distress with regular hygiene activities such as washing/brushing hair, brushing teeth, cutting finger/toe nails or hair or getting dressed.

- Avoid any sort of messy play or they will actively seek it out.

- Seek out, or avoid, rough-and-tumble play.

- Vary in tolerance for touch, to the extremes, from one day to the next.

- Resist/avoid certain sorts of fabrics, which makes getting dressed a struggle.

- Display distress when people are too close.

- Show an unusually intense need for certain textures, such as blankets, carpets, sweatshirts or other items. For example, my daughter constantly rubbed her pillow case and needed it in a specific position for her to feel right.

- Strongly resist putting hands in certain textures, such as sand, pumpkin guts, finger paint, glue, stickers, slime toys, etc. Or they may seek out such sensations.

- Insist on wearing socks at all times to avoid touching surfaces with feet or, alternatively, resist wearing socks to feel surfaces.

- Be particularly affected by textures of food.

- Squeeze in between furniture, couch cushions, tight-fitting places or ask to be hugged hard, squished or leaned on. My daughter hated being hugged, but she loved to be squished or squeezed.

- Feel calmed when joints or muscles are pressed on or massaged.

Certainly this list isn't exhaustive and symptoms vary from one child to another. There were times, for example, when my girl wanted me to bear hug her so hard that I was afraid of hurting her. Then on other days, she wanted me to do our 'Touching Game', where I lightly ran my forefinger over her limbs and torso. (This exercise is discussed in greater detail in Chapter 4.)

What parents need to know for now is that when the tactile system isn't functioning the way that it should, it has a huge impact on many everyday life activities such as eating, eliminating, social interaction, personal hygiene, affection, playing and so many other areas.

As a mother, the most painful thing to endure was not being able to comfort my child with my touch. Touching her only made things worse. It is heartbreaking to watch your child writhe in discomfort or fear and only be able to console her from afar.

But that's why we're setting up the Sensory Diet, so we can learn what our child's needs are at a given time. Then we can help our child up close and we can teach her that such sensations don't have to be so scary.

Proprioceptors: Coordinating Ourselves in the World

As mentioned earlier, this system helps us relate to the world around us by giving us information about our position (how far away or close we are to objects or people), movement (how our muscles help us move), gravity, head movement and balance. This system is divided into two areas: vestibular and proprioceptive.

Vestibular

This is the 'gravity sense' that tells the brain about movement. This sense tells the body whether we're moving or not and what direction we're going in. The vestibular system is also in charge of our coordination, balance, understanding gravity and muscle tone and it helps us to feel safe in our environment.

This system works closely with the auditory system to help us with balance, coordination and head movement. It also relies on the visual system to assist through eye movement, tracking and focusing. Both of these systems also work together with gravity to help us stay in an upright position and balance our bodies. Receptors in the inner ear pick up messages about gravity from the world around us, then tell the body how it should be moving or whether we are balanced the way we should be.

As with other systems, children can be over- or under-responsive to vestibular stimuli or they can bounce back and forth between the two, depending on what their bodies need at a given time. When this system isn't functioning properly, not only does balance and coordination seem 'off', but vision may also be affected. For example, they may have difficulty focusing on moving objects or they may struggle trying to read. They may also have trouble with learning language, speech and writing.

There are several characteristics that indicate vestibular dysfunction. The following list combines potential indicators of intolerance of movement, gravitational insecurity, under responsiveness, seeking and posture problems.

If your child experiences difficulty with his vestibular senses, he may:

- Avoid activities that involve rocking, swinging, spinning, sliding or going upside down. Such children may become anxious about recess or gym. Alternatively, he may crave continuous movement such as hanging upside down, spinning or sliding and never seem to get dizzy or bored of such movement.

- Move slowly and cautiously and avoid taking risks that may cause injury.

- Be terrified of heights, even if it's only the height of a curb or stair, and scream whenever he's lifted up.

- Be frightened by elevators and escalators.

- Be greatly dependent upon a trusted adult to help her with most physical activities or chores.

- Be fearful when another person tries moving her body or tipping her backward (e.g. swimming or washing hair).

- Seem obsessed with keeping environments and the people in it the same way.

- Need intense movement like jumping on the couch/bed, spinning in a swivel chair, staying in an upside-down position, stomping feet or spinning around on the floor on his knees.

- Be unable to feel when her body is falling and not try to protect herself from injury.

- Show difficulty with maintaining balance or refusing to take part in activities in which he doesn't use both feet at the same time, such as riding a bike, standing on one foot, doing jumping jacks, etc.

- Have what's called a 'rag doll' or 'wet noodle' body when picked up. The muscles seem to have low tone.

- Have a loose hand grip and show difficulty with using pens/pencils, scissors, eating utensils, brushing teeth, etc. Alternatively, she may handle objects with too much pressure to make up for not being able to get a good grip. (Does she press too hard with pens/pencils? Squeeze the family pet too hard when holding it?)

- Tire easily during activities or outings.

- Have poor gross and fine motor skills.

- Struggle with games requiring him to cross his midline (some examples would be 'Simon Says' or song/movement activities like, 'Head, Shoulders, Knees and Toes').

- Struggle with carrying out activities requiring many steps or with absorbing things they've just learning in order to be able to go on to something else.

Children with severe vestibular issues may even display poor self-esteem and social skills because they tend to avoid playground activities or games that make them uncomfortable. Or they may play games with so much enthusiasm that it intimidates peers. My daughter used to give up right away when she wasn't able to do something. She also got extremely agitated in new situations and worried excessively when an event was coming up that she knew might cause her some discomfort.

When my kids were younger, we got a computer dance game for them. It is similar to the popular video games of today, but this one plugged into the VCR and was geared for younger children. There was a mat with arrows pointing up, down, left and right and the child had to step on the correct arrow sequence when they saw it appear on the television screen to 'beat' the game. My daughter seemed excited about the game at first and wanted to try because she loved both music and dancing. But once the game began and the arrows scrolled up, she wasn't able to watch the arrows, coordinate her feet and stop at the right time all at once. Her body seemed to get all tangled up, then she crumpled in a ball on the floor, crying, and said, "I can't do it, Mama! There's too much to do. My feet aren't listening to my eyes."

On the one hand, I felt so sorry for her because after trying her best; her younger sister did the game more easily, laughing when she missed. But on the other hand, how smart of my daughter to realize what had happened! And the Sensory Diet is exactly what you need to help those feet work with the eyes, ears and other body parts to play such games more successfully.

Proprioceptive

This system helps tell us what our bodies are doing, keeps our body parts working as a team, gives us information about what our muscles and joints are doing and how much force we need to use to perform certain tasks. One description I love is from Carol Stock Kranowitz who said that the proprioceptive sense is our "internal eyes". It's in charge of reflexes, our automatic and planned reactions to things and self-awareness. It also allows us to gauge how close we are to something or someone and where our bodies are positioned in our environment. The system takes information from joints and muscles and helps us learn skilled movements.

Children struggling in this area have trouble coordinating their bodies to bounce a ball, play coordinating sports like baseball or hockey or take part in other activities like ice-skating, which can easily lead to losing a sense of control over their bodies. They may struggle to play with toy parts appropriately and often appear clumsy and bump into things.

The proprioceptive sense also works closely with the tactile and vestibular systems to help us know how much force we need to use when writing with a pencil or crayons, to understand that a cup of juice is much lighter than a full backpack and to know how to hold our heads and bodies when we're in motion or how to move our arms and legs to run, catch/throw a ball or manipulate toys the way we're supposed to. It also plays a significant role in our emotional security in our world. If we aren't sure how something or someone will cause our bodies to react, of course we'll feel scared, worried, insecure or even withdrawn.

The following are several characteristics that can explain your child's struggles with certain events or activities. This list includes reactions for children who are over- or under-responsive, seeking specific activities, have poor discrimination, trouble with movement, posture and/or emotional security:

- Doesn't like moving and gets upset when forced to.

- Doesn't like or avoids activities requiring her to use her muscles, like jumping, running or hopping.

- Seems to have poor muscle tone.

- Likes to crash into things or seems to bump into objects or people on purpose.

- Stomps his feet while walking or walks on tiptoe.

- Likes tight-fitting clothes or seems comforted by being swaddled or wrapped tightly in blankets.

- Chews on things she shouldn't, such as clothing, string, pencils or fingers. She may also enjoy crunchier/chewier foods that require a lot of jaw motion.

- Seems to lack accurate body awareness or fine/gross motor control and/or coordination.

- Holds pens/pencils too tightly so they break or too loosely so they drop out of the hand after minimal use.

- Seems to break toys and other objects frequently (e.g.: doesn't seem to be aware of how hard they handle things).

- Displays poor posture and balance.

Children who struggle with their proprioceptive sense may prefer to stick to familiar activities that they've mastered and avoid new situations or activities. One thing we heard a lot was, "I can't *do* that!" before the child had even given something new a try. This can result in low self-confidence and self-esteem.

Interoceptors: What's Happening on the Inside?

There are very few SPD resources that discuss this sensory system because it is rather complicated and extensive. So we'll do a general discussion as SPD does affect it and vice versa. And speaking from my personal experience, my children experienced such a high level of anxiety from their reactions to sensory stimuli that affected every aspect of their lives, I needed to know what those reactions were doing to their insides...the parts we *didn't* see.

This system involves all body regulations, including the major organs such as the heart, lungs, liver and stomach, and also the systems these organs are part of (circulatory, elimination, digestion, etc.) as well as the chemical and hormonal functions that occur within these systems.

When I first started writing this book, I was asked why I'd include such a complex system in a book written for parents. As touched on above, I think it's important, at the very least, to understand how SPD impacts the functionalities of the organs and systems, especially how the 'fight, flight or freeze' reaction interrupts the body's regular functions (see the sidebar, 'The Interoceptor System: The Connection to Anxiety and Panic Disorders' at the end of the chapter for more information).

When most of us are nervous, anxious or, especially, scared, our bodies go into a survival mode called, 'fight-or-flight'. Essentially this means that the body interrupts the normal way it works to make us more alert, aware and ready for action. The heart beats faster, breathing rate increases, digestion slows down, elimination slows down and the sensory systems are at peak performance. We become ultra-aware of smells, sounds and other sensations. To make all of this happen, hormones and body chemicals (such as cortisol, adrenaline and norepinephrine) shoot out into our systems. Once the event that caused the negative reactions is over, our body slows back down and gets us back into a calm state again.

However, if the body stays in a fight-or-flight state for an extended period of time, there can be negative consequences. Cortisol, for example, isn't bad for us in short periods of time and in small doses. But when people worry or are anxious most of the time, an excessive amount of cortisol pumps through the veins forcing the body to work overtime. This can be damaging to the organs and systems because they are forced to be on the alert all of the time, with no down time. Plus, the inability to calm down interferes with sleep patterns, eating, elimination and proper brain functioning.

Children with SPD, who are already on sensory alert, can experience this fight-or-flight response for most of their day, putting their little bodies through too much stress. This is the physiological side of SPD, what the physicians can most likely detect. The reason parents should be aware of the fight-or-flight state, and what negative impact it can have on the body, is that these physical reactions are testable, measurable and logical. This mistakenly becomes the focus of treatment when, in fact, it's the underlying *cause* for these reactions, a poorly functioning nervous system, that needs to be treated. It's unfortunate, but often parents are advised to put their children on medication to ease these reactions, even though this may not be necessary and does not address the underlying cause.

For example, my daughter was also diagnosed with severe anxiety in various areas (social, separation, general as well as obsessive-compulsive disorder [OCD]). When she was three-and-a-half, I was 'strongly advised' to consider putting her on an anti-anxiety medication and antidepressants. Having researched the issues, I knew there were other options I hadn't tried. The medication may have eased my daughter's overt symptoms, but her nervous system would have still been disorganized.

Knowing about, and understanding, the interoceptors and the fight-or-flight reaction is important because all of the systems are connected. When the brain can't deliver messages, the body doesn't understand how it's supposed to work and it becomes distressed. This distress puts the body into a fearful panic mode, ready for action (or reaction) at every moment. Although it's not necessary for parents to understand the minute details of all of the organs and hormones involved, they do need to understand their child's reactions so they can help him come back down to a state of inner calmness and, eventually, teach him to recognize for himself when he needs to do this.

The Sensory Diet helps all of these systems function properly and, eventually, it gets the brain, sensory and body systems working together as a team so the child can focus more on enjoying the world around him rather than worrying about how that world makes him feel.

The Interoceptor System:
The Connection to Anxiety and Panic Disorders

From a parent's perspective, one of the more devastating aspects of SPD is the anxiety it can cause the child. For example, before my daughter was diagnosed with SPD, she would become so fearful of the outside world that she refused to leave our house on most days. And it wasn't just the sensory stimuli she feared. It was more how those sensory stimuli made her body feel. She developed what's called *interoceptive fear*, with is a psychological term that means she was afraid of how her body reacted when it was stimulated. And it wasn't just when she was over-stimulated, as most children are from time to time.

But also, she didn't like how her tummy felt when she was nervous or how her heart beat faster when she wasn't sure about something or how her lungs needed her to breathe more when she moved too quickly. She didn't like the 'prickly feeling' on her scalp when the wind moved her hair or when certain touches on her skin gave her goosebumps. She put off certain activities, such as getting dressed because she knew certain clothes would drive her crazy. And she especially didn't like that when she ate or drank, she would eventually need to go to the bathroom.

When something causes us pain or discomfort, we avoid it. It's human nature and a basic survival skill. This is what can happen with children who have SPD. They don't like how something makes their body feel, so they avoid it. This is called *interceptor avoidance* and it's one of the main symptoms of panic and anxiety disorders because fear and avoidance are overt behaviors that can be observed and measured.

My daughter's reactions to even the slightest amount of stimulation were severe, leading psychologists to conclude that she had severe anxiety and OCD exclusively, not realizing where the fears stemmed from. I didn't deny that she had these fears. I just knew that in order to ease her anxieties I need to help her face the stimulations in a way that was fun, safe and calming.

When psychologists use "Exposure with Response Prevention" to treat people who have anxiety and panic disorders, they use a method called *interoceptive exposure*. This is when a therapist exposes a person to his fears one baby-step at a time, with the long-term goal being to get the fear under control. For example, if someone has a fear of the outside (agoraphobia), the therapist would set up a plan to start the patient standing in an open door looking outside. When this becomes tolerable, he'd then have the patient stand out on the front steps for a bit. After that, he'd see if the patient would go out on the front lawn, then maybe for a walk down the sidewalk, and so on until the person reaches his ultimate goal of, maybe, riding a crowded bus or going to a sporting event without fear. The Sensory Diet follows a similar protocol in treating children with SPD.

A child who refuses to be exposed to certain stimuli is disorganized and fearful during much of her day. An OT trained in the Sensory Diet and experienced with treating children with SPD help expose the child to the sensory stimulation she's afraid of slowly and gradually in a way that includes what she loves and is good at. Once her body learns that those sensations aren't so scary, she learns not to panic when her body feels those sensations. The end result is that she'll be able to come into contact with the once-feared stimuli, understand what her body's reactions will be then know which tactics she needs to use to reorganize herself.

That's why the Sensory Diet is so important for children with SPD and why early detection, assessment and treatment are essential. Without intervening in that fear and avoidance pattern, children won't be able to enjoy their lives to the fullest. And the longer they go without treatment, the more intense the fear becomes and the more difficult it is to treat them.

<table>
<tr><td>

3

</td><td>

So, What Exactly *Is* the Sensory Diet?

</td></tr>
</table>

Now that you have a solid understanding of how a nervous system and the various sensory systems are supposed to run, you're ready to jump in and learn about the Sensory Diet: what it is, who's involved, how it works and how it's set up.

Becoming 'Sensory Smart'

The term 'sensory smart' is used frequently by authors Lindsey Biel and Nancy Peske. It describes the level of understanding you must reach in order to be able to recognize when your child's sensory issues are causing her problems and when she needs help. Let me explain.

There were times when my daughter sat on the couch trying to watch a video, only to break into tears after about ten minutes. Until I really started paying attention, I didn't realize that her frustrations stemmed from being unable to concentrate on the video with all of the other things going on around her at the same time. The patio door was open, blowing the curtains around, allowing outside noises to flow in. Her younger sister, being only a baby at that time, was playing or trying to touch her. I may have been working or doing housework at the same time. The list goes on. One day, I decided to watch my daughter from a distance for a few minutes or, as my friend Lori says, "Watch her with sensory glasses on," in order to figure out what was truly going on.

As soon as I put her video on, she ran over to her favorite spot on the couch. At first, she seemed fine. Then she started rocking, hitting her head against the back of the couch. After a minute or so, she pushed herself up onto her hands and knees, rocking back and forth. She rocked for a couple of minutes in that position, then got up and walked around on the couch cushions. After pacing back and forth on the couch for a few more minutes, she finally flopped face down, covered her ears and exploded into tears.

That was my *"aha!"* moment when I realized that sitting still was difficult for a child whose body wanted to stay in constant motion, even when all she really wanted to do was watch a favorite movie or show. Plus, in my daughter's case, her little eyes darted around the room constantly as her attention was grabbed away at every second.

I now understand that her actions and behavior were her attempts at focusing her attention, but then she would break down because no matter how hard she tried or what she did, she still couldn't make herself concentrate on what she wanted to. My daughter knew that she needed something to help her in such situations, and that's how she was showing it. We just didn't have the right sensory tools, knowledge or understanding to help her back then. But we learned over time.

Once I became what Lindsey Biel and Nancy Peske, co-authors of the book *Raising A Sensory Smart Child*, call, 'sensory smart', I understood what parts of her diet she needed at what time so she was able to concentrate better on the tasks or fun-time activities at hand. The key is to be as in tune with your child as you can so that you develop this same level of understanding.

The Basics of the Sensory Diet

When a child struggles with dysfunction in sensory integration, he can have a really hard time concentrating on one thing. Think about it. Isn't it difficult to concentrate on what someone is saying to you when there's loud music blaring or other people talking to you at the same time? Wouldn't you find it distracting or irritating if a person was poking you or rubbing against you continuously while you tried focusing on a task? Or how frustrating it would be if you tried standing up, running or even maneuvering around objects only to fall down or crash into everything? A properly planned Sensory Diet, created with the combination of sensory knowledge from an experienced occupational therapist (OT), together with the inside knowledge about the child from his parents, helps provide the sensory nutrition his body needs *when he needs it most*.

An internationally renowned OT, Patricia Wilbarger, coined the term, 'Sensory Diet' in 1971. It refers to creating a daily schedule of specific sensory exercises individualized to a child's abilities and needs. Wilbarger included the word 'diet' to stress the importance of sensory input to our bodies in order to survive and thrive, just like our bodies need food and water.

This diet has more to do with 'feeding' the nervous system through activity, movement and sensory input, with an important nutritional element added in. You can think of it as a way of feeding your child's nervous system the necessary sensory input that isn't being digested properly on its own.

An OT works with the child's parents or caregivers, or other people involved with the child's therapy, to choose the exercise and activity options best suited to his needs as well as to determine how often, for how many minutes and how intensely the exercises should be done.

According to the American Occupational Therapist Association (AOTA), a well-planned Sensory Diet needs to have a good mix of exercises that include comfort touch, deep pressure and muscle stimulation, pleasurable social experiences, exercises that organize proprioception as well as varied tactile activities and modulating vestibular input. Finally, good nutrition, including extra doses of vitamins, minerals and 'brain friendly fats' (omega fats), while eliminating foods with artificial colors and dyes, as well as dairy and gluten rounds out a good Sensory Diet.

Important note: I can't stress enough how important it is for parents to seek the assistance of a professional in setting up a proper Sensory Diet. Believe me, I tried doing it all on my own and although it was possible, I missed some important elements that my daughter needed because I wasn't knowledgeable enough to see that her vestibular and proprioceptive systems were also out of whack.

Before her later SPD Occupational Therapy/Integrated Listening System (OT/iLs) program (discussed in later chapters), I did a lot of the exercises with her that I had found outlined in books and tried various therapies. I couldn't understand why she'd only progress to a certain point then revert back to where she was before we'd tried anything at all. I finally understood that it was because until I had her re-assessed by an OT specializing in sensory integration, I had no idea how poor her vestibular and proprioceptive systems actually were and how those systems were starving for sensory input too.

I'd been focusing so much on helping her with tactile, eating and more obvious sensory issues I had overlooked that she was clumsy, had terrible balance, couldn't do exercises or activities requiring her to use both sides of her body at the same time and that she struggled with understanding things consisting of more than two or three steps and other areas. It took the expertise of her new OT to see all of those things for me before I could *finally* get her on the right track.

The point is that parents really do need the help of an OT who is trained and experienced in working with children and adults with sensory integration issues. Such an expert can look at the child through more therapeutic lenses to be sure nothing is missed. Having that extra insight is crucial for setting up a successful diet. Plus, having the additional support is so comforting.

Who's Who in the Sensory Diet?

The major players in the Sensory Diet are an OT, a pediatrician and/or natural healthcare provider, a nutritionist and, of course, the parents. Each of these individuals brings a separate invaluable piece to the Sensory Diet team and together, they create the best possible base for your child's success.

The OT: The Main Connection

The OT is usually the person who creates a program for your child as well as trains parents how to manage the Sensory Diet at home, at school and in the community. The OT is also the one who assesses your child's sensory needs and provides advice on what specific activities he needs.

The role of an OT, as defined by the American Occupational Therapy Association's *Occupational Therapy Profession—Scope of Practice Definitions* (1994), is to help individuals improve their lives and well-being through, "purposeful activity or interventions designed to achieve functional outcomes, which promote health, prevent injury or disability and which develop, improve, sustain or restore the highest possible level of independence." In other words, you'd go to an OT when you are having difficulty functioning in your environment in an effective way.

These wonderful people teach life skills, such as dressing, cooking or eating and they can assist with social functioning skills. For example, they can help if you suffer with anxiety or other social disorders and they can help those who have physical barriers learn new ways of working and living in their environments. They can help with behavioral issues and even work with adults at work or children in the classroom to assist with specific needs.

When searching for an OT, there are specific things you should look for and ask about. Shop around and take the time to research your top choices. Set up an initial one-on-one meeting with the person so you can get to know her a bit and also describe your child's specific needs and your goals for him.

Here's a list of specific questions to ask at your initial meeting:

- *What is your specific training and experience?* You want a person who is not only trained and/or educated as an OT, but who also has several years of experience and is licensed. This is an important question to ask because a person who has only taken workshops or seminars on the subject of SPD will not be as helpful to you and your child as a person specifically trained in sensory integration, SPD, the nervous system and what to watch for. The OT who finally made a difference in my daughter's life, Kathy Mulka, trained at the S.T.A.R. Center with Dr. Lucy Miller and she, in turn, is training her assistant OTs with the same methods. That's about as top-notch as you can be.

- *Do you work with children and, if so, what age groups have you worked with and for how long?* This is just as important to ask about because a person may have loads of experience but if he has rarely or never worked with children, he may not have the level of understanding or patience that a person who works with children a lot would have.

- *What specific areas will you be working on with my child?* You'll want to know whether this person will just conduct the diagnostic part then suggest someone else, if she'll work on your child's complete sensory integration needs or just parts of it (for example, she may not address the eating or anxiety issues) and what other options she may have to offer you (e.g.: other forms of therapy for your child, support for the family, community support, etc.)

- *Will my child's therapy be conducted at your clinic or somewhere else?* My daughter's first OT sessions were done weekly in our home. Her new therapy sessions were conducted in the office where her initial assessments were done, using the same equipment she became familiar with during her assessments. It's important to know how the therapist likes to do her sessions and whether her style will work for you and your child.

- *What support do you offer parents/caregivers?* The whole family goes through the SPD journey together, so ask what sorts of options they may offer to help you cope too. After all, strong, knowledgeable and informed parents make the best advocates.

- *What experience do you have, if any, working within the school system?* The reason to ask this question is that there are many people in the school system who don't know about, don't understand or who don't 'buy into' SPD. Therefore, you need someone who understands how the school system works to help you get the support you need and to ensure that your child gets the assistance she needs in the classroom. A sensory-friendly classroom helps to keep children with sensory issues on track and ready to learn. An OT who is knowledgeable in this area can not only inform the school but also teach you how to advocate for your child's needs in school and in the community.

- *What are your fees and how do you bill?* Unfortunately, SPD therapy and treatment sessions aren't always covered under insurance plans because there's no 'code' for SPD... *yet.* (Insurance companies assign a numerical or alphanumeric code to each sort of disorder, disease or illness being treated as well as the sort of treatment being used. If there's no 'code', then there's little or no coverage.) This can be an expensive venture for families who don't have coverage or can't get it. The last OT my daughter had was very accommodating as she had many years of experience dealing with insurance companies. Never be afraid to ask what can be done, as most therapists just want the best for you and your family.

These are the main questions to bring with you when you're interviewing OTs. But never be afraid to ask any and all questions or bring up concerns. You'll be making an important investment – financially, emotionally and mentally – so you want to be sure any potential worries or problems are addressed at the front.

Lindsey Biel has some wonderful tips and advice on her Website, www.sensorysmarts.com, regarding choosing the best OT and other questions to ask. It also has some checklists you can print off and take with you.

The Health Provider: Physical Support

The health provider is the person, usually a doctor or nurse practitioner, your child sees to make sure her overall health is good and that nothing else could be contributing to her sensory issues. You most likely already had this person on board before seeking the guidance of an OT. It's not uncommon to need a physician's referral to get other assistance covered by insurance or to get OT services in school. But you can certainly seek out an OT on our own without the referral.

It's essential that your healthcare provider, whether a traditional physician or naturopath, is supportive of what you're doing for your child's sensory issues. Most doctors only want the very best for your child's overall health and work with you to help him. I only mention this because there are, sadly, some physicians who aren't supportive of the concepts of SPD. This is strictly due to the lack of understanding or knowledge, and they sometimes try steering parents in an entirely different direction (e.g.: suggesting a mental health practitioner or focusing more on behavioral issues). This only puts more stress on you and, indirectly, on your child so if your child's doctor isn't supportive, either inform her as best you can or find another doctor who specializes in, or has experience in, treating children with SPD. The less stress on your shoulders, and the more support behind you, the better.

Here are a few points that your doctor needs to be kept in the loop about:

- Updated reports from your child's OT, or any other therapist, on treatment options, progress and other information. If everyone is on the same page and communicating well, then the child has the greatest chance for success.

- Be sure to have the doctor give you written reports that you can add to your OTs file on any colds, flus, allergies or other illnesses your child experiences as well as how such illnesses are being treated. I didn't realize until my daughter began her therapy with her new OT that when these children have a cold, like any of us, it effects how the vestibular system (balance, muscle agility, etc.) works as well as how it communicates with the other sensory systems. All of the sensory exercises OTs use tap right into this system because they're trying to strengthen it. So, when a child's system is already weakened from cold or flu, tapping into these systems only drains them further, resulting in him seeming even more sensitive, grouchier or exhausted than usual. For that reason, have your physician keep the OT updated and have the OT keep the physician updated on all treatments. Better still, reduce the intensity of vestibular input during colds or it could result in an adverse reaction. This is discussed further in later chapters.

- If during a session your OT observes something about your child's physical health that has less or nothing to do with his sensory issues, have her make a specific report for your physician. That way, the doctor can do a thorough physical examination and determine whether any other tests should be carried out.

Overall, the physician's part of the Sensory Diet is to be the 'body' of the mind-body-spirit connection that is essential to overall health. Keep him informed, provide him with OT or other therapy reports and embrace his pearls of wisdom regarding health issues.

The Nutritionist: Feeding the Hungry Brain.

I've found it extremely helpful to have someone whose expertise I can tap into about essential 'brain foods' as well as what to include / eliminate from a child's diet. Of course you can get the basic information on nutrition from your healthcare provider, but an experienced pediatric nutritionist who specializes in children with neurological disorders can definitely help provide you with additional information on how to feed your child's hungry brain.

All children need a healthy nutritional balance of vitamins, minerals, proteins and fats for overall brain functioning and health. Such nutritional elements are critical for children with SPD. "The nervous system is 60 to 70 percent fats, so the fat you eat literally becomes your brain," says Kelly Dorfman, Licensed Dietician Nutritionist (L.D.N.). "Studies have proved that the kind of fats you eat change the way your nervous system works. You need other nutrients to metabolize and utilize fats properly and for other neurological functions. Therefore, your nutrient availability affects your brain functions. Period. And if the nutrition situation is bad enough, you cannot learn."

A nutritionist can help in the following ways:

- Educate parents on what foods and combinations of specific foods will help their child the most.

- Educate parents on 'brain-friendly' eating.

- Set up a nutritional plan, including what foods to eliminate and what foods to include. They can even help parents figure out how to get the same nutrients from different foods. This is necessary for the tactile-sensitive child who is a fussy eater. It gives parents foods with different textures to choose from.

- Help parents understand how to read labels and avoid foods with artificial dyes, colors and flavorings.

- Teach families which foods can trigger specific negative reactions, behavioral issues and even produce certain overt behaviors that may be mistaken for symptoms of other disorders (e.g.: ADHD, autism spectrum disorder and others).

- Teach families living on a budget how to feed their sensory-sensitive child in the most effective way without breaking the bank.

- Teach parents how to advocate for their child's hungry brain in school and in the community.

Parents: The Glue of the Team

Parents understand their child better than anyone. It only makes sense that their input would be crucial to the Diet's success. You're with your child all of the time. You know what sets him off, what worries him, what freaks him out, how he'll possibly react in certain situations and what he needs in order to calm down. Therapists need your input in order to understand the child, his interactions, his reactions to the home exercises and his part in the family dynamics. What these people see in therapy rooms can be very different from what you see at home.

As a parent, you see your child more from a protective, loving and emotional standpoint, whereas a therapist sees her in terms of what the best route is to helping her function better in the world around her. If you're able to shed some light on what she likes, what she doesn't, what makes her 'tick', etc., it can help the OT get closer to her and find common ground to start and work from.

Here's what parents can do to contribute to the Sensory Diet team:

- Provide the child's history, including pregnancy, birth and infant development.

- Give insight into the sorts of sensory-seeking or aversions the child has and what sorts of things he does to cope with it.

- Describe what the child is like during the course of the day, including the times she's 'up' or 'down'.

- Give insight into things like sleeping and eating patterns, social interaction and how the child relates to siblings and other family members.

- Offer insight into what works and what doesn't in terms of exercise suggestions in the Sensory Diet so the OT knows what to work on.

- Help the child in the community by taking what is learned in therapy and teaching others.

In addition to these major players, your child may also need the help of speech therapy, feeding OT (if the OT you work with doesn't work on this side of things) and, possibly, a behaviorist to help with dealing with such issues as communication, tantrums, discipline etc.

How is the Diet Set Up?

The way an assessment is conducted varies depending on a child's history, current treatment and any other concurrent conditions your child has. Generally, though, the assessments for sensory needs are relatively similar.

Assessments are usually done in two one-hour sessions so as not to overwhelm the child and so the OT can focus on one specific area at a time. With my daughter's therapy sessions, for example, I went in twice. During the first visit, her fine and gross motor skills were tested through fun-time activities like drawing, sorting pennies, coloring, handling balls and moving activities for her arms and legs. The point of all of these activities was to test things like eye-hand coordination, direction/steps, fine motor muscle agility and to check for signs of dyspraxia (e.g.: whether she gets 'lost' doing tasks with several steps or if she struggles with crossing objects over her midline).

During the second visit, she got to go into the sensory gym where the focus was on her gross motor skills such as balance, following directions/steps and tapping into her proprioception abilities by getting her to climb, swing and balance.

During this portion, the OTs watch for things like:

- Ability to organize her body to do a set task.

- Muscle strength.

- Balance.

- Threshold for things like touch, her body leaving the ground, holding a pose without getting tired and moving her body in space.

- Moving all of her body parts at the same time or coordinating both sides of her body to do a specific task (e.g.: passing a ball from one hand to the other, jumping, running, getting her body to weave around things without bumping into them, doing a movement like a somersault, etc.).

- Understanding and carrying out a task with more than two steps.

- Her need or lack of desire to move.

- Walking on her tiptoes, indicating a need for vestibular input (e.g.: weight).

Most times, children don't even realize they're being observed or tested because the OTs use activities that are fun but that require the child to be able to move her body in a certain way. How she carries out the task, or her inability to, tells them what sensory systems aren't functioning properly.

While all of this is going on, you, the parent, complete various sensory questionnaires to indicate what your child's sensory sensitivities are in the home, at school and in the community. Once the OT records all of her observations, combining it with the child's history and sensory-questionnaire responses from the parent, she analyzes the information and makes recommendations for treatment. The goals of the initial therapy are to figure out the exact exercises the child needs, enjoys and responds to as well as to train the parent(s) how to carry out the same sensory exercises in the home.

What our daughter needed the most, for example, was to learn to tolerate touch so I could do her deep-pressure touch exercises, tolerate things like standing on wobbly or unbalanced things to get her proprioception input, tolerate specific weight-bearing exercises to get her vestibular input and how to connect words to her feelings to let us know what she was feeling and for self-regulation. In addition to this, I was participating in 'Parent Ed' where I was given lessons on SPD, suggestions for how to help her at home and tips on what to do for her at school.

After our five weekly sessions, her OT created a wonderful Sensory Diet including what sorts of exercises she needed at what times, when and for how long.

Our Diet consisted of things like this:

- *Tasks for auditory regulation:* My daughter freaked out in situations that were too busy and loud, with too many sources demanding her attention. This, as I found out, stemmed from her auditory deregulation and her inability to distinguish different pitches to determine what was, and wasn't, a threatening sound. Kathy suggested a good set of headphones to block out sounds she didn't need to pay attention to in order to focus.

- *Regular vestibular input:* More heavy jobs. Kathy said the fact that my daughter walked, ran and did just about everything on her tiptoes was a sign that she needed extra weight in order to feel organized. She instructed me to do vestibular exercises, or 'heavy jobs', every 60 to 90 minutes to help her stay calm (see Chapter Six for suggestions).

- *Regular proprioceptive input.* When a child has a disorganized proprioceptive system, she needs exercises that strengthen balance and ease fear of movement or leaving the ground. My girl needed to do at least two types of exercises per session (usually after school or first thing in the morning), such as doing fun activities while standing on a wobble board, swinging, spinning, balancing on a T-stool or climbing onto a small stepladder and jumping into a pile of pillows. All of these exercises tap into the proprioceptive system and, at the very least, help the child feel less anxious about what her body does and how certain movements make her feel.

- *Tactile stimulation.* Children who are tactile-defensive need to be gently exposed to certain touch sensations in order to learn how to cope with them in the future. When a child is protected from experiencing sensations they fear, the problem may get worse.

- An example is that my daughter's tactile defensiveness was so bad at times that she wouldn't touch anything with her hands or do things that got them dirty or even put her hands out to stop herself from falling because she didn't want to feel anything. She was *that* anxious with how things made her feel! Now, that doesn't mean we should grab a child's hand and shove it into pumpkin goo or make him finger-paint when his body isn't ready for the sensation. It means we introduce him to things slowly by preparing him for that sensation, then give him tools afterward to calm down from how that sensation makes him feel.

- Kathy suggested that since my daughter was extremely sensitive to light touch, and felt better with deep touch, I should do activities and crafts that have different textures in order to keep her aware of such things, but then have 'feel good touch' exercises such as her Pizza Game, Sandwich Game, Rice Box, bear hugs and similar tactics to calm her down (see Chapter Five for more details).

- *Help with dyspraxia: Organizing the outside world organizes the inside.* For many years, I knew my daughter struggled with the ability to understand instructions with a lot of steps, and that she had a strong need for sameness as well as a need for visual cues. She had a tendency to get 'lost' when performing a task with too many instructions and would literally do it over and over, her frustration rising with each re-do, trying to get it. I never had a word for this condition until she saw Kathy: *dyspraxia*.

- Kathy suggested that I give my girl a lot of visual cues, explain things to her in a step-by-step way, with very small numbers of steps, and then do lot of prompting. My daughter's way of holding on to the familiar and trying to get the rest of us to stick with what she knew and understood was how she tried staying organized. She got little charts and pictures and was able to understand what she needed to do next and when.

- *Working through emotions.* Children with SPD often have poor emotional development. Helping a child connect to how things make her feel is so important. This teaches her, 'Hey, when that person bumps into me, that scares me, but I can _____ instead of scream and cry.' It isn't that she doesn't feel. It's more that her body is so disorganized that she isn't able to understand how things really make her feel.

- Kathy suggested I discuss feelings with my daughter so she learned to understand things like happy, angry, sad, scared,

lonely – what makes her feel those things and what she can
do to work through a feeling that gets a bit too big for her.

The point of the Sensory Diet is to learn exactly what your child
needs in order to feel more organized and able to cope in the world
around him. Some parents may feel strange doing the exercises or are
uncertain whether they really help. I was told to think of it this way: If
your child had a disease, such as diabetes, you'd need to understand
what your child needed to help her get through the day. This may
include an organized schedule of exercise, blood sugar regulation, eating
properly, shots, etc. When such a child is running around like crazy
and, seemingly out of control, she may need a shot to bring down her
glucose level. If she's lethargic, she may need a sugar/nutrition boost.
Your child has a disorder that requires constant sensory stimulation at
specific times to organize her brain and nervous system. Her exercises
are her 'medicine' and she depends on it to get her through her day.
That's why the setting up of a Sensory Diet is so important.

As your child grows and changes, his sensory needs, and, therefore,
his Sensory Diet, also changes. If you ever find that your child isn't
responding to the exercises the way she used to, see your OT for an
update and suggestions for tweaks to the Diet. Eventually, your child
will be able to regulate herself and know exactly what she needs. Until
then, she depends on you.

The Wonderful World of Alternative Therapies

Many parents of children living with sensory issues seek holistic, natural
ways to treat their child. The following is a list of fabulous natural and
holistic forms of treatment that have been known to help children with
SPD and sensory issues. Note that not every treatment works for every
child, so be certain to choose what suits your child's current needs,
research the practice thoroughly, find the best therapist in that
treatment area and then give it a try. Sometimes trying a combination of
different forms of treatment works the best. Don't be discouraged if it
takes a while to figure out what works for your child. Take your time
and keep trying until something 'clicks'.

Chiropractic

The focus of chiropractics is to address abnormal movement of nerves,
muscles and joints. It can also help with posture and teaches the child to
be more aware of her movements within her environment. Chiropractic
neurologists can be of particular help because they assess and

rehabilitate brain imbalances. A fantastic resource on this subject is Dr. Shane Steadman's website, http://integratedbraincenters.com/about/. Dr. Steadman believes the key to treating children with neurological disorders is re-connecting the mind and body by defragmenting the nervous system. In other words, the child must learn to be aware of her body and what it can do, without fear.

Craniosacral Therapy (CST)

In short, craniosacral therapy involves assessing how well the child's craniosacral system works, which means the therapist checks the effectiveness of the membranes and fluids that help to protect the brain and spine. All that's done is light touch massage on the bones and structures of the skull. It's supposed to help correct the adverse results (such as sensory, motor and neurological dysfunction) stemming from imbalances during the development of the brain and spinal cord. A great resource to learning more about this procedure is Dr. John Upledger's website, www.upledger.com (recommended by Carol Stock Kranowitz). Please check out www.craniosacraltherapy.org. Many parents report being pleased with the results of this therapy.

Hippotherapy

This horseback riding therapy can help posture, movement and sensory processing. Essentially, OTs as well as physical and speech therapists integrate movements of horses into regular therapy interventions. One mother in my group said it did wonders for her son's muscle tone, reaction to stimulation and sensory-motor skills. A great place to find more information is the American Hippotherapy Association's website, www.americanhippotherapyassociation.org.

Perceptual Motor Therapy

The idea behind perceptual motor therapy is to get the child to participate in activities stimulating left/right brain integration so he learns to be more in tune with what's happening to the nervous system when he does things. It's very effective for children whose body aware-ness is fairly poor and who struggle with performing tasks requiring the use of both hands, crossing over their midline or using both sides of the body at the same time.

This form of therapy can also help with balance and coordination as well as help the child learn new ways to cope with the sensory informa-tion he comes in contact with.

Physical Therapy

These therapists help to improve a person's physical ability. For children with SPD, they encourage activities that help to strengthen muscular control and motor coordination so the child can prepare his or her muscles for movement.

For more information or therapist recommendations in your area, visit the American Physical Therapy Association (www.apta.org) or the Canadian Physical Therapy Association (www.physiotherapy.ca).

Integrated Listening System (iLs) Training

Dr. Alfred Tomatis, an eyes-ear-nose specialist, realized that by targeting specific areas of the brain using 'filtered' music and music with different pitches and tones, it was possible to retrain and improve sensory, motor and learning processing. Most specifically, he realized that music helped improve the functioning of the brain stem and cortex. The founders of iLs, Kate O'Brien Minson and Randall Redfield, built on Tomatis' realization. They found that by using movement in conjunction with the music they could help integrate sensory information much more effectively.

The idea behind iLs is similar to that of listening therapy except that the headphones or iLs are specially equipped with a tiny piece called a 'bone conductor'. The way we hear our own voice is very different from how others hear it or how it sounds on a voice recorder. Essentially, the bone conductor lets us experience sounds in '3-D' or in a more pure form. Not only that, but the person participates in activities while listening to the iLs program as a way to get their visual, auditory and vestibular systems working in sync. For people, especially children, whose sensory systems have never been integrated or working together, the world can be a terrifying place.

Another significant difference between iLs and other 'listening programs' is that iLs has developed a Sensory Motor Program specifically for SPD and autism spectrum disorder. It is based on years of feedback from therapists working with this population of kids and it uses frequencies in a way that is completely different from the Tomatis programs.

In summary, the sound waves created during iLs training create electrical impulses in the inner ear that are passed along to the brain. It's these impulses that help us to learn to focus and concentrate on what we need to. People whose brains aren't getting enough of this vital 'energy' such as those with SPD or ADHD, don't have the same ability to pay attention, focus or tune things out the way they're supposed to. The child wears headphones and listens to the specialized music while doing play or OT. The key is to get all of these sensory systems working together. You can learn more about this therapy at the iLs website, www.integratedlistening.com.

Reiki

The practice of Reiki, a Japanese concept, is most often translated as 'Universal Life Energy'. It's a non-manipulative healing art using our life energy. It began in Japan in the late 1800s with Mikao Usui, who developed the original Reiki system of healing. In 1930, Hawayo Takata brought Reiki to the Western world. Today, there are literally hundreds of different Reiki systems being taught and practiced with a variety of corresponding philosophies about the healing art. Reiki is a healing technique based on the principle that the therapist can channel energy into the patient by means of touch, to activate the natural healing processes of the patient's body and restore physical and emotional well-being.

This form of therapy can help children with severe tactile defensiveness because it gets the child to focus on her body's energy and, as Karen Gordon says, it, "softens distractions [so] the child can experience a certain degree of calm or support or relaxation." Learn more about the Reiki practice on these websites: Karen Gordon (http://revivehealingarts.com/karen-gordon/), The International Center for Reiki Training (www.reiki.org) or the Canadian Reiki Association (www.reiki.ca).

4 Sensory Integration Through Play

> Play Therapy is based upon the fact that play is the child's natural medium of self-expression. It is an opportunity, which is given to the child to 'play out' his feelings and problems, just as in certain types of adult therapy an individual 'talks out' his difficulties.
>
> ~ Virginia Axline, psychologist and creator of Play Therapy

As discussed throughout this book, children living with SPD need help organizing their bodies and integrating the sensory messages that are trying to get through. The way to do this is by introducing them to sensory stimulation through gentle and gradual exposure. This can be a very scary experience for children who actively avoid sensations that they perceive as 'hurting' them. But by using fun activities, games and crafts geared to your child's needs, likes and abilities, she'll be more willing to try those 'scary' activities and will barely notice that she's in therapy!

Now, your immediate thought might be, "How can play help my child cope with his sensory issues?" Those were my initial thoughts too. But I learned that play is actually used by many therapists who work with young children for several reasons:

- It's a 'middle ground' where the adult comes down to the child's level and comfort zone.

- It paves a smoother path for getting a child to open up because the adult is tapping in on activities the child likes.

- It gives a therapist a way to interact with a child without having to intimidate her with 'scary' questions.

- It helps a child 'talk' about issues she normally wouldn't because she's initially using toys or objects to 'speak' for (or

through) her instead of directly talking about a troubling
issue.

- It gives children with communication difficulties a way to
  'talk' to others.

- The way a child plays and interacts with toys or objects can
  tell an observer a lot about the child and his needs, which
  gives direction for approaches in therapy.

For further reading on the rationale of play therapy, I recommend
Schaefer's *Therapeutic Power of Play* (2013).

Play gives therapists an amazing way to introduce new sensations, or
sensations your child actively avoids, in a safe, fun way. For example,
some children with sensory issues can be extremely tactile-defensive and
actively avoid specific sensations that involve touch, being touched,
getting dirty or, most of all, getting sticky/messy/sparkly/fuzzy stuff all
over their hands. These children tend to walk around with their hands
clenched in fists to avoid contact with anything that could cause
discomfort. Incredibly, OTs can instill courage in these children to try
out things they never have before such as using glitter glue, finger
painting, playing with shave cream, tolerating different fabrics against
their skin and even allowing much-needed joint and muscle massages.

So how are OTs able to encourage our children to give such activities
a try? The therapist works with the child to get her past her severe
sensitivity to light touch in order to get her to the deep pressure she
needs by introducing the sensations to her while she is doing an activity
that she enjoys. By the end of this chapter, this strategy will be clearer
to you. You'll also have answers to other questions you might have
including: What kinds of therapy use play and what are the differences
among them? What is the point of using play? How do OTs determine a
child's specific sensory needs and how does play help target those
needs?

Understanding the purpose of using play to help sensory integration
gives a parent the insight not only into why they're doing the exercises
they are with their child at home, but also how to put exercises and
games together in the most effective way for the child's Sensory Diet.

In addition to discussing integrating the senses through play, this
chapter includes suggestions for using play in the Sensory Diet at home
and at school.

Play Therapy vs. Sensory Integration Therapy

Although many forms of pediatric therapy use play in at least part of the sessions, there are basically two main forms of therapy specifically using play that children with SPD may encounter: play therapy and sensory integration (SI) therapy.

Play therapists and SI therapists are similar in that both forms of therapy are child-centered. What this means is that the child is given a great deal of control, or at least made to feel that they have control, in terms of the direction the therapy sessions take.

Control is something children often feel like they lack, so having the power of choice helps ease a great deal of stress and tension for them in a therapeutic setting. Having choices may also help many children with severe sensory issues, who often don't feel any sort of control over what happens to or in their bodies or how their bodies react to stimulation, feel less threatened in the new environment of the sensory gym. (The sensory gym is where OTs usually conduct SI therapy. It's filled with swings, gym mats, crash mats and fun toys and equipment.) Having the power to choose certain activities he enjoys or feels safe doing can be a great ice-breaker, while also giving the therapist a place to branch out from.

The main differences between the two forms of therapy are the therapist's training and how he chooses to use the play in his sessions. The chart in the next section of this chapter outlines a few of the main similarities and differences between play therapy and SI therapy.

Similarities and Differences

Play Therapy	SI Therapy
Therapist usually has an educational background in psychology or psychiatry or other mental health field with emphasis on child psychology and/or early childhood development. They are also Registered Play Therapists.	Therapist is usually an OT, or has occupational therapy in addition to other education, with extensive training in the nervous system, sensory issues (specifically SPD), the sensory systems and how to tap into these systems.
Therapist uses directive or non-directive forms of play* (depending on the child) to change or encourage a behavior or to help work through a stressful experience.	Therapist is highly interactive with the child ('plays' with him). Therapist uses fun games, activities and exercises to stimulate sensory systems in order to help the child learn effective ways of coping with those sensations. Focus is not so much on

	behavior as it is retraining the brain to understand sensations and to help organize the nervous system.
Unless the therapist wants the child focusing on a specific behavior by using certain tools, sessions usually stem from what activities the child chooses and are child-directed. (e.g.: My daughter usually stuck with the sandbox, Mr. Potato Head and things she could do with her 'beanie' Tigger.)	Sessions are highly structured and guided by the therapist but based on the child's interests and needs. (e.g.: My daughter's favorite sensory exercise was 'crashing' so her OT worked that into the session with other activities.) Therapists usually let the child choose a favorite activity, or take turns with the child choosing activities (e.g.: My daughter's turn, Kathy's turn, etc.), then manipulate the activities so the child also gets tactile, motor-planning and other sensory stimulation at the same time.
Therapy can be individual, parent/child, family or group, depending on the child's needs.	Sessions are most often conducted with the child alone. However, if the child's social development needs extra work, there could be sessions with another, or few other, same-aged children. The therapist may also have a caregiver or siblings participate in parts of sessions to learn techniques for at-home exercises and one-on-one counseling with caregivers to answer questions, discuss strategies and learn how to advocate for their child in the world.
Play therapy may be covered by insurance plans (especially when part of early intervention strategies) when incorporated with psychological, early intervention therapy or other traditional forms of therapy.	If categorized as 'occupational therapy', some of the sessions can be covered under insurance plans, but in most cases, SI Therapy or SPD OT isn't covered at all, leaving parents paying out-of-pocket. Integrated Listening System (iLs) or other non-traditional forms of therapy are also often not covered.

Directive therapy is when the therapist leads the therapeutic process. In play therapy, for example, the therapist chooses specific activities, games or toys to help a child focus on a certain behavior or emotional experience. *Non-directive therapy* allows the child to take the lead. The therapist may reflect back the information the child is providing, either verbally or non-verbally, but the child initiates the direction of the therapy session.

As you can see, both forms of therapy stem from the same basis: child-based therapy using play through which to 'communicate'. But it's the SI therapy that children with SPD are usually set up with and from which their sensory diet is designed. I feel it is important to understand both main forms of therapy that use play because there are times, as in our case, when a child may need to do both, or one before the other, in order to feel comfortable getting started.

My daughter, for example, had a very tough time when we first attempted the SI therapy with an OT. There could have been many reasons for her agitation and struggles, but we thought it was because (a) the therapy was conducted in our home, her 'safe place', then she had no separation between the two; (b) something about Donna, her first OT, triggered negative sensory stimulation for my daughter that she wasn't able to handle at that time; or (c) her body just wasn't ready to deal with both the therapy and the social interaction at the same time.

To this day, I haven't been able to pinpoint exactly what it was that caused her reactions, but I felt that in order to prepare her for the SI therapy her body needed, I had to get her ready for the interaction part of the therapy first. She had severe social anxiety on top of her sensory issues. This was mainly because she was never sure who, or what, would make her body feel 'bad', so she learned to fear other people, places, animals or toys that she wasn't sure about.

If this is the case with your child, it's probably a good idea to have your child begin with a form of non-directive play therapy, then try the more intensive SI therapy.

Play Therapy: A Good First Step

The form of play therapy that we began with was perfect for my daughter at that time. It was child-focused and nondirective and she was allowed to choose the activities and toys she wanted to play with, and her play therapist taught me how to interact with her using those toys and activities.

The therapist advised that the parent isn't supposed to ask the child any questions or direct the play in any way. Parents are merely supposed to give the occasional interjection (e.g.: "Oh! Tigger loved to swing!" or "The cat is under the sand."), then wait for the child to include the parent in the play. This sounds simple enough, but it can be difficult for some caregivers to get used to the format at first. After all, the natural thing for us to do during play is to ask questions or try getting right in there and helping to steer the play in other directions. That's what makes playing so fun, right?

Allowing the child to direct the play gives him the opportunity to 'tell' you things that are on his mind without him feeling pressured to answer questions. Play therapy doesn't even require verbal language in order to be effective. Plus, for children with more severe sensory or social issues, undirected play therapy gives him a way to play with others in a manner most comfortable to him until he's ready to go further. After a year or so, my daughter learned to tolerate people speaking around or to her, then, eventually, even tolerating others playing *with* her. By the end of her sessions, she even allowed her siblings and me to actively participate in her play.

Another way that play therapy can help children with sensory and social issues is that parents learn how to play with their child as well as how to use play as a positive way to work out what their child feels. For example, my daughter never spoke much and usually only gestured or pointed. Play gave her a voice and her toys gave her a way to show the rest of us how she felt or what she wanted or needed. It was a blessing. What parents might find, however, is that play therapy alone doesn't address sensory issues directly.

Play therapists either try to reduce an undesirable behavior or teach a desirable one through play. So, even though the therapist may help the child with the overt behavior or reaction to sensory stimulation, the intolerance to the sensory stimulation is still there. And if that intolerance isn't dealt with appropriately, it can worsen. A neural connection needs to be made so the child not only learns to experience that sensation without fear, but also learns how to cope with it.

Plus, play therapists don't usually deal with any additional issues related to SPD, such as dyspraxia, which is generally recognized to be an impairment or immaturity of the organization of movement. Associated with this may be problems with language, perception and thought, or vestibular or proprioceptive needs.

That's what SI therapy does.

SI Therapy: Play That Addresses the Sensory Side of Things

In SI therapy, the focus is less on the behaviors the child is displaying and more on where that behavior stems from. The therapist's view is that if you dig to the root of the behavior or reaction, which for our sensational kids is their need for proper sensory input and under-standing of that input, the behavior or reaction lessens dramatically.

As mentioned in Chapter 2, the first step in SI therapy is to take a full sensory profile to assess your child's sensory needs. The results of the assessment, combined with information from a parent consultation, lay the groundwork for your child's program.

With more sensitive children, it's best to start with a component that causes the lease amount of stress then slowly add things. For example, aside from my daughter's sensory issues and dyspraxia, she had different sorts of anxieties, the most prominent ones being social and separation. On her first day of OT, Kathy allowed me to stay in the room the entire session. When I joined them for the next session, Kathy said, "We're going to get Mom to watch a video in the next room while we finish playing, okay?" There was no video, of course, but it helped my daughter feel better knowing I'd still be close by, even if I wasn't right there with her.

After a few sessions, I didn't even go in the room. Kathy simply asked, "Would you like Mom to come with us, or will you be okay on your own?" And my daughter said, "I'll be okay". That was a big hurdle for her to overcome, and once she was able to go into the gym alone, not worrying about where I was or what I was doing, she was able to allow herself to focus on the next hurdle.

SI therapy is highly interactive and your child's therapists will give her constant positive feedback to encourage her to keep trying things she's struggling with or to go a bit further in an area she's already comfortable in. Feedback may include high fives, clapping, patting, a deep-pressure rub or even just a, "Hey! You did it! Good for you! Let's try again." Children thrive on this sort of external feedback, especially for children whose sensory issues may make them feel such activities are impossible for them. What's most important with SI therapists, however, is that they teach the child to do things because they feel good rather than just for the high fives or verbal rewards which becomes reinforcing in itself.

After a while, the therapist may start asking your child things like, "So, how did that make your body feel?" or "What did you like about that?" or "What can we do to make it even better?" Such questions demonstrate the key to this form of therapy—getting the child to be more in tune with his body so he learns what he needs at what times to calm his body down or to bring it back up.

Another aspect that makes this form of therapy effective is that the therapist works with the child in a sort of baby-step format. Therapy starts with the least threatening form of a certain sensory stimulation then works up to the level the child needs. For example, if your child struggles with vestibular issues, the therapist may want to have her use a swing to get used to that sensation. Different kinds of swings are used (tire, hammocks, rings, etc.) so if your child is very defensive with such a stimulation, he may start with the least 'scary' form, perhaps a hammock. While in the hammock, the therapist explains what the swing is doing and asks the child, "How's that? Do you want to go higher/faster/slower? How does your body feel when I do _____? (The therapist may 'bump' the swing or change the direction or move from back and forth to side to side, etc. This simulates different sensations and may feel differently in the child's body.)

From there the therapist may have the child play little games using that swing, maybe the Fishing Game (see Chapter Six). Once she seems comfortable with the 'safer' swing, the OT may do the same game using the platform swing with an inner tube on top of it and leaning out to catch the fish, etc.

What's the point? Introducing sensations in baby steps and introducing similar stimuli in different ways:

- Introduces the sensation.

- Allows the child to 'feel' what that sensation does to his body.

- Helps him learn words to describe those sensations.

- Helps him experience the same stimulations in different ways, as he would in the 'real world'.

- Helps him figure out how much, or how little, his body needs that sensation.

- Helps him learn ways to cope with that sensation.

- Helps him feel successful.

This baby-step approach truly eases your child into areas you may have never thought he'd venture. And when you mix this baby-step approach with encouraging interaction, and the child's active participation in his therapy, you have a recipe for success. The child is not only learning to feel comfortable with his body and how the world around him makes it feel, but he's also learning valuable social, organizational and coping skills. And this is all going on without him realizing that it's 'therapy'.

Your child will feel safe in SI therapy because there is someone besides her trusted caregiver who 'gets' what she's going through. That connection allows her to be led into sensory areas she is normally scared to tap into. But, as explained, your child's therapist always begins with the safest area for your child, adding what she needs slowly as her comfort levels rise, until she *asks* for that stimulation on her own. (Yes! That *will* happen!)

Let's say your child's favorite thing to do is to jump and 'crash' onto the foam mats. In order to get the proper sensory input into other sensory systems, the therapist may get your child to navigate through an obstacle course that includes jumping, balancing, throwing, squeezing through a tunnel *then* ending with crashing on her favorite foam mat.

On my daughter's first day, Kathy respected some of her more sensitive areas, such as tactile and started earning her trust by having her choose her 'safe' activities, such as crashing and jumping. Even though they didn't ask her to touch and feel things, she still engaged in tactile exercises (e.g.: handling different textured balls during a swinging activity), but she accepted this as part of the fun stuff she wanted to get to. So you see, in SI therapy the child still gets to choose some of the activities she wants to do, but the OTs tweak those activities so she's still getting the level of sensory input she needs and can handle at one time.

Another great aspect of SI therapy is that the therapists often do the activities *with* your child. Modeling is so important for our kids, especially when they have vestibular, proprioceptive and dyspraxia (motor-planning) issues. To learn planning and how to follow steps or rules, they may play a game of baseball or Swing Bumps (see Chapter Six), once he isn't nervous about the movement of the swing, and keep score. Or try a game of Scooter Board Bowling (Chapter Six). These are all games that tap into specific sensory systems while teaching things like social skills, being friends, playing fairly and understanding and remembering steps and rules. Such games also help teach children how to be a 'good sport' and to let go of the idea that they always have to win.

Not all children have to go the route of using the play therapy approach before starting SI therapy. But, it's helpful to know about both so that you can determine which might be a better fit for your child in terms of what she is able to handle initially. It's also good for parents to note that there are play therapists who focus on children with sensory issues, but parents need to ask the therapist whether they have specific sensory integration training. Additionally, parents have to ascertain whether the child and the therapist are a good fit for each other or therapy may not work. For more background, see *Play Therapy: The Art of the Relationship* (Landreth, 2012).

Why Is Play Important to Sensory Integration?

Okay, so you've learned what the forms of play therapy are and why play is important, but why is it important specifically in SI therapy? In addition to the general points listed earlier, and the discussion of SI therapy above, play is vital in SI therapy for the following reasons:

- *Play introduces the child to sensations she otherwise avoids.* If your child has severe tactile issues, for example, she most likely avoids any sort of touch sensation that she isn't that she isn't comfortable with. That can make life very difficult to enjoy. Having your child play games that introduce various textures or forms of touch can help her get past those 'light' touches that may drive her crazy to allow the more 'heavy or deep' touches she actually likes and needs.

- *Play teaches her how to get the stimulation she's seeking but may not be doing it in the most appropriate ways.* 'Seekers' actively seek out sensations but may not be doing it in the most appropriate ways. For a child who has high olfactory or gustatory needs, for example, going around smelling and tasting everything isn't always safe because he could get sick. SI therapy, instead, teaches him games or activities using specific tools (such as chewy toys or different textured foods for oral stimulation or 'smelly' games for olfactory input) as well as introduces him to sensory tools he can carry around that give him that needed stimulation.

- *Play teaches motor-planning.* Some children with SPD struggle with planning out how to get their bodies to coordinate for an activity. Maybe your child gets 'stuck' when climbing on a climbing wall or she doesn't seem to understand rules in a sports game or he isn't able to coordinate his body to play 'real life' Wii games. These children can learn these skills through playing simple games that teach their brains to make the important connections that are necessary for moving both sides of the body at the same time.

- *Play increases self-confidence.* Kids who have convinced themselves that they 'can't' do things suddenly find that they *can* because the activities are geared to their needs and likes.

This confidence helps inspire them to try other things and not fear the new as much.

Additionally, SI therapy confers additional benefits:

- *Strengthens fine and gross motor skills.* As you've learned in earlier chapters, children with SPD commonly have weak muscle tone, tire easily in activity and struggle with things like writing, holding pencils, knowing how tightly or softly they hold objects or how hard their feet hit the ground. My daughter, for example, walked around with her toes curled under the balls of her feet. Essentially, she walked on her toe joints! She could sit, stand and even run like that. It hurt my feet just watching her. As I learned through her OT, there were two reasons she walked that way: (1) she needed more vestibular input, and (2) she sought more muscle and joint stimulation (proprioceptive). It actually took that much pressure for her to 'feel' those sensations.

- SI therapy gets these kids playing games wearing weighted vests, carrying heavier objects around the gym, squeezing through tent tubes and doing other fun activities to 'feel' their muscles and joints and to get the heavy input their bodies crave. Plus, they get to draw, string beads, make crafts or play games like Operation that help to work on fine motor skills and eye-hand coordination.

- *Helps children with dyspraxia.* Children with dyspraxia tend to get 'lost' when performing activities that require several step-by-step instructions. During therapy, OTs help your child learn visual cues, visual planning and other handy coping methods to get them through their day.

- *Improves the child's eating.* Often, one of the major concerns for parents with sensitive children is that they don't eat much. Whether it's their child's sensitive palate or their olfactory or tactile systems. OTs can help introduce children to different types of foods in fun ways and get them back on track with eating.

From my personal experience, play and SI therapy have given my daughter three things she'd never had before: (1) a connection with her environment and a slowly growing courage to explore it, (2) 'sensory tools' to help her cope in a world that was often filled with too much sensory stimulation and (3) a spark of confidence that grew with each baby step she took.

By now, the statement quoted from Kathy at the beginning of this chapter should be crystal clear. Play gives us a way to 'reach' and 'reach out' to our child in a fun, safe way and introduce her to new sensations in ways that are fun, safe and familiar. The next few chapters describe and discuss many of those fantastically fun activities.

Learning More about SI Fun

The purpose of this chapter is to ease your mind about what happens when you let go of your child's hand and watch him to into the sensory gym with his therapist. Letting go can be difficult because you are so used to caring for your child's needs yourself. Initially, it can feel hurtful when you see another person interacting with and 'reaching' your child in ways you have never been able to. Believe me, I understand.

These wonderful OTs aren't trying to do things better. They are merely trying to give your child the strength, courage and knowledge to live her life the way she deserves to, without fear or pain. Learning about this process is important because knowledge gives you a much broader understanding of your child's struggles and how you can help her through them.

During our daughter's sessions with Kathy, I was given a lot of information that I never had before. I viewed videos of other parents going through what I was, but how they developed the tools to truly care for their child's needs at home. I was empowered and enlightened by our OT's amazing knowledge of SPD. Not just what it is, but also the physiological, emotional, social and mental sides of the disorder. And, most importantly, I learned the best way to help my child through hands-on methods. I never let a day go by when we didn't practice her sensory diet or teach her how to get through tough transitions or to cheer her on to keep going when her world was too overwhelming and scary. We need to absorb knowledge from as many sources as we can.

Many books are out there from people who 'get' what our children need. But don't take the books and follow them verbatim. Take the author's tips and mix them into what you're already doing. Learn a new exercise and put your own spin on it so it fits your child's specific needs. Once I started doing that, and making the activities fun 'family time' instead of simply 'therapy time', my daughter responded better, she progressed further and we, as a family, became closer than ever.

5

Exercising Your Child's Exteroceptors

The focus in this chapter is exercises, tips, strategies and tools to stimulate your child's exteroceptors. I'll have suggestions of what to try for each sensory system in this category – taste, smell, hearing, sight and touch. Before I delve in, I need to cover two important points.

First, always refer to your child's own tailor-made sensory diet before taking on any of these suggested exercises. Your OT will outline what your child needs, and when, based on her own sensory sensitivity levels, so use my suggestions only as a guide, working them in where they'll help the most. Remember that trying to do exercises meant to stimulate when your child is already over-stimulated may result in the opposite effect of what it's supposed to do.

Because my daughter was both a 'seeker' and an 'avoider' (and this could change from one hour to the next), we had a wide variety of activities we used with her. This chapter also tells you where you can purchase specific tools or how you can make your own version of the tools whenever possible.

As you are likely aware, your child may be very uncomfortable trying some of these exercises at first. My daughter could be so tactile defensive that even thinking about someone touching her caused her to become anxious or want to avoid an activity or the person entirely.

As mentioned in earlier chapters, it's a natural reaction to want to protect your child from discomfort and, I'll admit, I'd allowed my daughter to avoid things too. But if I continued allowing her to avoid the things that made her uncomfortable, she never would have learned how to cope with those tactile sensations, and that was crucial for her overall functioning in the world.

Second, only do what your child can handle at any given time. That means when she comes home from school, she may not want to go zooming around on her scooter board. Instead, she may need to curl up on the couch under her weighted blanket and 'zone out' for a while. Or he may want go into his swing or to his 'calm down place' until he gets rid of the extra stimulation from the day at school. And, as you probably already know, what your child needs on one day may be very different the next. Just try something out and if she reacts negatively or pulls away, don't push it. As mentioned earlier, if you push something just because it's on her schedule, or because the books tell you to and it's not what her body *needs*, you could throw her into immediate overdrive and she'll be out of sorts for the rest of the day or evening.

It's okay if something doesn't work at first. Take baby steps and applaud every effort. I'll give you many things to try, including ways to calm your child down afterward.

Sidebar: Snoezelen Rooms

Years ago, when we began creating a place for my daughter that was 'sensory friendly' (a place filled with all of the tools she needed to get the input she needed and when), I had no idea there was a technical name for such a place. A Snoezelen Room (see www.snoezelen.info for more information).

Snoezelen rooms were created by Ad Verheul and Jan Hulsegge in the early 1980's. They created the name from the words 'Suffelen' (meaning to seek out or explore) and 'Doezelen' (to relax). These are the main things we are trying to help our kids do. The original Snoezelen rooms were to offer a quality recreation and relaxation experience for severely disabled adults.

Verheul and Hulsegge felt that Snoezelen rooms should be self-directed by the patients. They also believed that the idea of Snoezelen offered users the freedom to make their own choices. Clients can react and respond to the sensory stimulation in these beautiful worlds in their own special way, which is also much of the basis of the Sensory Diet. The purpose of these rooms is to stimulate the user's sensory systems in a manner that feels safe, comfortable and fun.

Because these rooms are created with children and adults with sensory and neurological issues in mind, they are rich in sensory stimulation and help the brain to create, strengthen or repair neural connections. Some of the important benefits of such places include:

- Stimulates the seven senses.

- Serves as an excellent addition to regular therapy options.

- Provides a safe environment for kids to practice their Sensory Diets in.

- Helps increase functionality, awareness and attention.
- Helps improve memory, cognition and speech.
- Helps encourage movement, range of motion and posture.
- Teaches and encourages social interaction.
- Decreases aggression and anxiety.

When creating such a place for your child, it's important to ensure to include these six components:

1. **Soothing sounds.** Create your child's sensory space in a quieter part of your home, away from all the regular hustle and bustle and distracting noise. Include calming music or nature noises in the space or room that your child enjoys.

2. **Intriguing aroma.** Many doctors who treat children with neurological disorders or other conditions, such as ADD or ADHD, use scents or essential oils for a calming effect. Of course, if there are scents and aromas that your child already finds calming include those in their space. Some of the more popular choices include:

   o **Lavender.** This oil is known for its calming and sedative effects. Rubbing a few drops on child's feet, shoulders or chest can help him relax and sleep more easily.

   o **Cedarwood.** Considered a 'healing oil', it is high in sesquiterpenes, which is one of the chemical compounds that help to stimulate brain function and mental synergy. This oil can be applied on the forehead and neck, inhaled and massaged at the base of the skull near the brain stem.

   o **Vetiver.** This one is lesser known, but its musky aroma seems to calm over-energized kids while increasing attention and concentration. Small children may want or need only to smell it, while teenagers and adults can apply the oil gently on the shoulders or neck.

   o **Frankincense.** This is often used for mental, emotional and spiritual healing. Some research has shown it has been used in conjunction with other therapies for people who've suffered from brain injury, emotional and physical trauma and with those living with learning difficulties to improve their mental function.

3. **Interesting light effects.** Traditional Snoezelen rooms contain a variety of lights including string lights, bubble or lava lamps, globes and other visually stimulating forms of light. If your child is more sensitive to light, have such lighting in the room but start with a gentle form of light (e.g.: dimmed or natural light) then gradually introduce them to other forms of light.

4. **Comfortable seating.** Include different forms of seating, such as bean bags, rocking or foamy chairs. We also have body pillows, various textured cushions and a huge blow-up cushion.

5. **Choice of sensations.** This is essential for a Snoezelen/Sensory room. The whole point of such a place is to introduce your child to different forms of sensory stimuli in a safe, calm environment. The calmer his body is, the more willing he will be to experience the world around him. Be sure to have a wide variety of tools, toys and materials to tap into all seven senses. (There are many examples in the previous and next several chapters.)

6. **Opportunities for interaction and engagement.** Even though play in the room should be self-directed and your child should guide what sort of sensory input he's ready for, always be close by to help find opportunities to interact and engage your child in the space. You don't necessarily need to ask her questions, just add in little phrases here and there to let her know you're 'with her'. "Those string lights are beautiful." Or "I never thought to use that fidget that way. May I try too?" or "I see you smiling while you smell that pillow. Did you notice that it has different 'feels' too?"

   Here are some resources for Snoezelen/Sensory rooms:

   • Flaghouse (www.flaghouse.ca) is a course of many tools, toys and equipment.

   • Innovaid (http://innovaid.ca/) is another Canadian company that offers a great selection of weighted/non-weighted and constrictive items.

   • Pocket Full of Therapy (www.pfot.com) is an online store offering everything from seat cushions, products for midline issues and more.

- Southpaw Enterprises (www.southpawenterprises.com) offers a wide variety of products for many different levels of needs including sensory issues. You can get everything from fidgets to jungle gym equipment.

- Therapy In A Bin (https://therapyinabin.com/we-heart-canada/) a wide variety of supplies for your sensory sensitive child and they deliver to Canada!

Exercises for the Auditory System

An important point to remember when doing exercises to help your child's auditory sense is that just because he can *hear* sounds doesn't mean he *understands* the sounds. The auditory sensory system is deeply connected to the visual and vestibular systems so, usually, when helping the sense of hearing, it's wise to use exercises that involve all three senses, or try to. Movement is so important to the auditory system because it helps connect to the sounds being made to how your child's body is supposed to understand and interact with them. Plus, as discussed earlier, head movement, equilibrium and other body movements that connect us to our world are helped by a well-functioning auditory system.

From my own children's experience, the three movement and music methods that have been most effective include iLs Therapy, Listening Therapy and BrainDance. Listening Therapy is similar to iLs in that the child wears headphones with specially programmed music, but iLs is done with vestibular input while Listening Therapy is done with more calming activities, so the child is really 'listening'.

BrainDance is a program created by Anne Green Gilbert, who is an author, dance instructor and educator. The program combines music and specific movements to help make and strengthen neural connections. If you don't have access to these therapies, creating your own system is the very best thing. Music, with its different pitches, tones, tempos, rhythms and sounds, is a fantastic way to help sensory sensitive children learn to distinguish and understand sounds.

Some of these exercises require music and instruments, which you can buy or build the instruments yourself. I've done a bit of both but with four kids in the house, we always needed extras.

Here's how to make some of your own musical instruments:

- *Drum:* Use a variety of pots, pans and bakeware with wooden or steel utensils. You can even have ribbon or string to tie around the handles so your child can wear it like a drum.

- *Tambourine:* Staple or glue tin or regular pie plates together with dried beans, rice, coffee or vanilla beans (for added olfactory stimulation) inside. You can also tie bells or other jingly items around the edges for extra noise.

- *Shakers:* Put beans, rice or small pasta inside tin cans and seal them shut with tinfoil and a rubber band. You can also use yogurt cups, toilet paper or paper towel rolls or Tupperware containers that seal well. Have your child decorate her shaker in her own style to make it her own.

- *Whistle/kazoo:* We actually used empty snack-sized raisin boxes. It sounds the same as blowing on a blade of grass between the thumbs. Try partially sealing the end of a straw or putting wax paper over a comb to make a wind instrument. Another idea is to blow up a balloon then slowly allow the air to leak out. This is fun and hilarious all at the same time.

- *Rain stick:* Seal one end of a long empty gift-wrap tube. Put a few handfuls of rice, tiny grains of gravel or sand inside then seal the other end. Your child can decorate the tube with markers, paint or stickers before setting it up.

- *Didgeridoo:* Use a gift-wrap tube and have your child blow raspberries into one end. Have your child experiment with the different sounds his mouth can make to sound like a traditional didgeridoo. Tip: Toilet paper and paper towel rolls can also make great oral instruments. Be creative!

- *Dance ribbons:* Use straws, smooth sticks, hangers or plastic rods with a long ribbon tied to one end. You can get ribbons of varying color, texture or thickness for very little money.

For the music, you can purchase a CD with different types of music or create your own mix. Some suggestions to include are any classical, opera, jazz or funky music along with kid band stuff like The Wiggles, Sesame Street, Baby Einstein or other music your child likes.

With instruments in hand, here are a few fun games to try with them:

- *Family Parade:* Have everyone dress up in a favorite costume or other clothing and march around the house making as much noise as possible. This is a fantastic 'seeking' activity because it's loud and kids are banging, shaking and blowing their instrument. 'Avoiders' may not like this game at first, so see if she is willing to do it with headphones on. After a few times, try to get your child to march in time to a beat.

- *Red Light/Green Light:* This is a great way to teach your child about rhythm and keeping time. It helps him 'hear' and understand different tempos and beats. Play your CD and have your child (or children) play along. When the music stops, they stop. When the music begins again, so do they. If someone continues after the music stops, he or she is 'out' until one person is left.

- *How Does This Music Sound?* Kids love the opportunity to express themselves, so put on your CD and ask your child questions like, "How does this music make your body feel?" or "What feeling does this music sound like?" Then ask him to move his body to how the music 'feels'.

- *Musical Copycats:* For this game Mom or Dad takes the lead by tapping out a rhythm or playing a short song, then having the child copy you. Another version of this is to start with a very short pattern, have the child copy it, then do harder and longer patterns until everyone is 'out'.

- *Rock-and-Roll Star:* For this, you simply put on a DVD or CD of your child's favorite kids' group, grab his favorite instrument (if he wants to use one) and go crazy! The best DVD choices are those with a lot of singing, dancing and movement. Some excellent suggestions include The Wiggles, Barney, The Imagination Movers or Elmo.

Of course, a good old-fashioned game of Musical Chairs can always be a hit too. It's great to have a variety of listening games to play because there may be days when your child won't be able to tolerate music or instruments but still needs their auditory input.

Here are a few additional suggestions:

- *Simon Says:* Many children with dyspraxia or issues with crossing over the midline may struggle with this game at first, but it is a great game for helping with such issues.

- *Do You Hear What I Hear?*: I used this game with both of my sensory kids. Depending on how many people there are, sit in a circle or just face each other and take turns making animal, household or other noises. Whoever guesses right gets to go next.

- *Guess What I Have:* One person hides an object in her hand or behind her back while the other person has to ask questions in order to guess what the object is. This is a great game for planning, memory and attention.

Exercises for the Olfactory System

It's actually easier than you'd think to incorporate 'smelly' stimulation into your child's Sensory Diet. If your child is like how my daughter was, he probably smells anything and everything but certain smells drive him into sensory overload such as a person's individual smell or certain types of food while they are cooking, which can also add to eating struggles.

The only caution I'd like to make is not to use your child's calming smells for therapeutic purposes. For example, my daughter loved the smell of vanilla (which she said her beanie Tigger smelled like) or our laundry detergent (which was unscented, chemical and dye-free and I couldn't detect a scent but she liked it). She also had a toddler-sized pacifier she loved smelling. These are things she found calming when she'd be 'up' so we kept those smells for that purpose.

On that note, I'll jump right into a few 'smelly' games and activities to add to your child's Sensory Diet.

- *P.U: The Guessing Game of Smells or Smelly-Sticker Board Games:* Several years ago, I found a fantastic board game called 'P.U.' All of my kids loved it. Each player chooses a little animal token to move around the board. Along the way, you land on 'Good', 'Bad' or 'Mystery' spaces where you have to draw a card, scratch it then try to guess what the smell is. If you are right, you go again. If you miss it, your turn is over. The first one to reach the end wins! If you can't find this awesome game, you can create your own version by buying different colors of cardstock paper for Good, Bad and Mystery smells. Dollar stores sell stickers fairly cheap. Find all the smelly ones you can and make up your own game board. We had both versions going in our house.

- *What's That Smell?:* This can be a fun game as long as your child is up for it. It's definitely best to choose a day when she's seeking and open to the stimulation. Cover your child's eyes with a blindfold or have her close or cover her eyes if she isn't keen on having something tied around her head. Then have different containers or baggies filled with different smelly items. Have a nice variety of strong, mild, pleasant, stinky and other smells to really stimulate those nose receptors. Some great suggestions are coffee beans, various herbs or spices, candies, pine needles, flowers, essential oils. Other ideas include cooked or sandwich meat, fruit, perfume, scented soaps or anything else around your home. Keep points and the person who guesses the greatest number of items correctly wins. Note: Be careful with essential oils as they can be very powerful and cause unpleasant effects. Make sure the ones you choose are safe and used for calming.

- *Scented Play-Doh:* When my daughter first tried working with smelly Play-Doh, she gagged and washed her hands until she couldn't smell it on her skin anymore. Eventually, she sought out smell in her play so after re-introducing it to her, she was more accepting. I made our own Doh with Kool-Aid or other brands of powdered drink crystals. My only side note on this activity is that the crystals often have artificial dyes, chemicals and flavorings so if you are following the Feingold Plan, or another special diet, you may want to try the recipe below, which uses natural food colors and things like cinnamon, essential oils or other natural smells.
  Tip: If you have a highly tactile child who doesn't like smells, color or Play-Doh residue on his hands, have antiseptic wipes or a bucket of water close by so he can always wash off his hands. Certain Kool-Aid colors can temporarily stain the skin so prepare your child for this ahead of time if need be and have the proper clean-up stuff close by.

- *Smelly Beanbag Toss:* If you're a crafty person, you can make different beanbags yourself with various kinds of materials, textures, colors and sizes. You can make the filling out of beans, coffee beans, rice, pasta or other items that have a scent of their own. Or you can scent them yourself as desired. For those who aren't quite as good with the sewing machine, you can buy beanbags in the toy section of most department or toy stores or even in sport stores. Then you can open them to add your scent, or a bit more weight if your child needs it. Then you sew it back up and you're good to go. You could also make a Beanbag Toss board with different sized holes, each hole worth a certain number of points. Other options are to use pots, Tupperware containers or bakeware of varying sizes and shapes.

Tip: You can add an element to the game by having the person guess or describe the smell before tossing.

- *'Guess What' Flash Cards*: All you need for this game is to get some cardboard or poster board cut up into card sizes. Then get all of the scratch-and-sniff stickers you can find to create some flash cards with them. Put a sticker on one side and the picture or 'answer' on the other.

You don't need to just play games to expose your child to different aromas. Take her to a greenhouse, a bakery or for a nature walk where smells from wonderful to stinky are all around her. Get her experiencing, talking about and describing different smells so she learns to cope with them.

Play-Doh Recipe

2 cups flour

1 cup salt

2 cups boiling water

2 tablespoons vegetable oil

4 teaspoons cream of tartar (optional)

2 packets of Kool-Aid, other drink mix or food color

In mixing bowl, combine flour, salt, cream of tartar (if you choose to use it). Add in boiling water and oil. Stir and add your coloring, then cool and store in an airtight container or baggie.

Exercises for the Gustatory System and for Oral Stimulation

The olfactory and gustatory systems work so closely together, you can actually combine a lot of these activities with those suggested for olfactory. You'll notice that when your child is trying to experience something, in addition to touching it, she may also smell the object then mouth it. My daughter smelled absolutely everything, especially if something was new. And she chewed on clothing, writing instruments, her bed frame, paper or anything that was in her hands. She didn't even realize she did it. Most of the time, children mouth things, or stick them in their mouths, (e.g.: sucking, biting, chewing, etc.) not necessarily to taste them, but more because they need the oral stimulation. And that's what these exercises help with. The bonus to having regular oral stimulation is that it can help with certain eating issues, such as chewing and swallowing.

The following are exercises and cool sensory gear to help your child cope with his oral stimulation needs:

- *Chewies:* These are rubbery chew toys specifically made to give your child's mouth muscles a good workout. You can think of them as a 'teether' for older children. They come in a variety of shapes, colors, textures and sizes. And some companies such as Kid Companion and its *chewelry* line even make them into jewelry or design them to fit onto the top of a pencil or pen.

- *Wind Instruments:* As mentioned in the auditory section, any instruments that your child needs to blow into, such as flutes, harmonicas, kazoos, whistles, etc., are excellent for oral stimulation.
  Tip: You can get kazoos that have fancy additions, such as rings, 'copters or little balls. When your child blows hard enough into the kazoo, the ring or balls fly up into the air. We had one that looked like an alligator's face with two little plastic eyeballs. When you blew softly, the eyes hovered above the eyeholes and when you blew hard they went flying in different directions. This toy provided many hours of hysterical laughter. Another version of this is a Magic Ball Pipe.

- *Blowing Bubbles:* Who doesn't like blowing bubbles? And you can use household items to create different sizes. In *Sensory Integration Therapy* (Arnwine, 2007) the author even suggests using large pop bottles or milk jugs.
  Tip: Blowing bubbles helps your child with breath control (understanding how much force is needed to blow bubbles), and working the mouth muscles (to form the mouth into an 'O' shape). Plus you can play our favorite game with bubbles. Blow and Pop. One person blows tons of bubbles and the other(s) have to pop as many as they can before the bubbles disappear. Or you could play a game to have one person blow a few bubbles while the other(s) try keeping them afloat.

- *BloPens:* These are little painting tools. Your child blows in one end, and paint sprays out of the other. There are different versions so be sure to choose ones that make your child work a bit to get the paint going, but not so much that they're feeling dizzy after a while.

- *Drinking Straws:* Who knew that a straw could be used for more than just drinking? Though drinking out of a straw is good for sensory children too, straws can also be used to chew on, blow bubbles (with bubble blowing solution or in milk), blow paint (put a blob of paint on paper then have your child blow it across the page to make a picture) or even play our Blow Balls game. Gather a bunch of small balls (like the small super bouncy ones), ping pong, plastic or golf balls then have our child blow them across the room using the straw. Try that game as part of a sensory obstacle course or as a race with siblings or friends.

- *Pinwheels:* These are fairly easy to find and very inexpensive. If your child likes them as much as mine did, it may be to your advantage to make them. Bonnie Arnwine offers a great pinwheel craft in her book. Pinwheels are an excellent oral tool because you must blow it in a certain way to get it to spin and the harder you blow, the faster it goes. It's also an instant 'reward' to have the pinwheel spin so your child knows she's done it right. Pinwheels can also have visual benefits, especially if the colors are contrasting. You can move the pinwheel around so your child has to adjust her head and/or eye position.

- *Party Blowouts:* There are so many varieties to choose from. You can get plain ones or ones that have fringes, curls or feathers. Some make horn noises too. You can even get fabulous two- or three-way blowouts these days, which I highly recommend if you can find them. You can find party blowouts at a dollar store or party supply store.

  Note: These are *not* recommended for chewing. They are usually made of paper, colored and/or dyed and are not good to eat. In addition, the ends are usually made of the cheaper plastic and can splinter when chewed. Younger children should be watched when using them.

- *Snacks:* Offer your child a variety of snack types: crunchy (Cheerios, nuts, crackers, popcorn), chewy (licorice, Gummi bears, gum) or hard (juicy or plain ice cubes, crunchy toast or croutons). Obviously you'll have to make some alternative snack choices if you're eliminating gluten from your child's diet.

Exercises for the Visual System

As with the auditory system, just because a child can see things, it doesn't mean that she understands what she's seeing. I figured out that the reason my daughter didn't make eye contact often was because she couldn't watch a person's face moving and actually hear what they person was saying to her at the same time. Some people's facial movements really freaked her out. Exposing your child to as many visually stimulating things as you can, tapping into patterns, colors, textures, movement, light/darkness, etc. is so important in creating the neural connections your child needs for those experiences.

Help your child find meaning in what she's seeing by introducing different versions of her favorite things to watch or look at. Some visual tools to have on hand include:

- *Books that make him 'look':* A great example is the 'Where's Waldo?' books or the board game 'Hunt and Seek'. A lot of children with visual discriminatory issues aren't able to find things, even when they're looking right at them, if there is a lot of visual stimulation around. These types of books and games help teach them to focus on the object they have to in a fun way. Another exercise is to ask your child to describe the emotions expressed on faces in a picture book.

- *Bubble or lava lamps:* These fun psychedelic items from the '60s and '70's have actually become a staple feature in many Snoezelen rooms around the world. See the sidebar in Chapter Five for more information about Snoezelen rooms, which are essentially 'sensory rooms'. It lists things to include in your own customized 'sensory room' and where you can find those items. Not only do these lamps provide visual stimulation but they also offer a great calming effect when you're playing your Pizza Game or doing other calming exercises.

- *Kaleidoscopes:* These tube-shaped tools have a hole in one end that your child can peek into. As she turns the end, your child sees different shapes and colors that change as she twists. You can still get these at your local toy store or science stores. Sometimes these can make a child dizzy watching the patterns switch. Simply remind her to take it slow and to enjoy the colors and patterns she sees. Maybe even get her to describe what she sees.

- *Magnifying glass:* For an avoider, this fun tool gives kids reason to want to look really closely at things. My kids liked to play 'Super Spy' and 'Hide-and-Seek' with it. You can get them at most dollar stores, toy stores or science stores.

- *Etch-A-Sketch:* Yes, they still make these. They're good for strengthening fine motor skills as well as visual skills. Ask your child to draw something, such as faces, shapes, patterns, animals or favorite food.

- *Water or sand toys:* Toy stores sell wonderful play sets you can use with water or sand. They have parts that spin, jump, make noise or other wonderful visually stimulating movements.

- *Dartboard games:* These are great for focus and eye-hand coordination. I got my kids a magnetic one from the dollar store (much safer than a 'normal' one). You can also find ones with Velcro. A great version of this game is decorating a Bobo doll like a coconut tree. Find some plastic practice golf balls and cover one side of them with Velcro and randomly put the other side of the Velcro on your coconut tree, wherever your child thinks a coconut should go. Then all you do is throw your 'coconuts' at the tree and try making them all stick.

- *Visual cue sets*: Many children with visual issues also have issues with dyspraxia. This is because the eyes aren't giving enough information to the brain about what they're seeing to tell the rest of the body how to organize, focus or how to get started on something. Visual cards, lists and stickers representing tasks or activities help to give these kids an edge.

Here are a few activities you can use as suggested or with some of the tools above:

- *Hide-and-Seek:* This game is the best, and least expensive, way to have your child learn to 'look for' something. Be sure to use a limited area for hiding object so your child doesn't get 'lost' or frustrated while searching. Some variations for this include Stuffy Hide-and Seek or Hippity-Hop Ball Hot-and-Cold (Hide up to five objects around a room and the finder bounces on his Hippity-Hop ball trying to locate the objects. As he bounces closer to an object, the hider said, 'Hot!' and if he gets too far away, the hider says, 'Cold!' This game gives some vestibular input too and gets your child practicing his ability to find one object within others). I would suggest saving Hide-and-Seek games for when your child is somewhat rested and organized. It requires a fair bit of concentration and patience, which your child may not have when he's tired.

- *Eye Spy:* This is a great game that can be played absolutely anywhere. Start with having your child find a pre-selected object described to her only by color, then color and shape, then color, shape and size, etc. What you're doing with this game is getting her to look for specific objects and also helping her focus on specific aspects of those objects. As with any 'look for' games, start with something easy then slowly increase the difficulty level.

- *Fishing:* This is a game that my daughter learned with Kathy. She'd sit inside an inner tube placed on top of a platform swing. Kathy then asked where she wanted to go fishing and swung her around as if her 'boat' were setting sail on the fishing expedition. Once in her fishing spot, my daughter used different 'fishing poles' to catch fish on the floor below. Her fishing rod (a pole with string tied to it) had a magnet on the end that caught fish with paper clips on their mouths. Using another fishing tool that looked like a long pair of barbeque tongs, she leaned out over the inner tube and grabbed the fish. Once she got all the fish, her ship set sail back home and she could decide whether it would be a short, smooth ride (low swings) or a long, bumpy ride (high swings). This version of the game gives the child vestibular and proprioceptive input as well as visual discrimination practice. You can tweak it to suit your child's abilities and needs. A company called Flaghouse sells a version of this game. It's a vest filled with weighted fish and a rod so your child can fish, then use the vest for the proprioceptive input.

- *Stack and Crash:* You can use blocks of any kinds with this (letters, colored or plain) or, as Carol Stock Kranowitz suggests in her book, *The Out Of Sync Child Has Fun*, you could use differently sized and shaped boxes. Pull them all out, have your child build them into towers or whatever she wants to then let her knock them all down. My kids loved to create little houses for their 'guys' (little toys they collected) and absorb themselves in imaginative play. My oldest called it 'making a movie'. For other twists, have your child sort them by shape, color or size. If you can find blocks that have textures as well, this adds another sensory element to the game.

- *Bouncy Coconut Tree:* Using the coconut tree idea from earlier, have your child jump on a trampoline while throwing the coconuts at the tree. Be sure to keep points. You can also use a Hippity-Hop ball version where you place the coconuts around the room, get your child to bounce over to them, then come back to the tree and throw them. Or you can use a balance board or yoga ball for him to balance on while throwing. Use the same suggestions for any dartboard game.

- *Visual Board Game Suggestions:* For those who want some family game suggestions to stimulate visual skills, here are a few of our favorites: Whack-A-Mole, Hungry Hippos, Ants in the Pants, Don't Spill the Beans, Barrel of Monkeys, Connect Four, Gator Golf, Guess Who?, Mouse Trap and Candyland. These are all games that will have your child looking, seeking, counting and watching fun things happen when they engage in interactive play.

Exercises for the Tactile System

I understand the difficulties and concerns that come with having a child who has extreme tactile defensiveness, therefore this section of the book is very close to my heart. I could fill an entire chapter with tips on coping with tactile issues. This section covers the most important tools and gadgets to have on hand and I'll also share some of the activities that worked best with my daughter.

She had huge struggles in this area. In terms of touch, she had been almost exclusively an avoider her entire life. She didn't like touching things or being touched, especially if it involved her hands or getting her hands dirty, sticky or messy. She couldn't deal with regular forms of affection, like hugs, cuddles, kisses or having her hair stroked, she only felt good in certain kinds of fabrics and avoided peers who were too 'touchy/feely'.

Touch doesn't just impact what touches your child or what he touches. It also influences what he plays with, who he allows to be close to him, what he eats, where he goes, what he sits on, where/when he eliminates and the list goes on. The tactile system, as you learned earlier, is greatly influenced by texture, temperature, weather (e.g.: wind, rain, snow, humidity), pressure and other stimuli that most of us don't even notice. It's usually a lighter touch that bothers children with tactile sensitivities the most. But in order to learn to function effectively in the world, you have to help your child experience tactile sensations so he can learn the best ways to cope with them.

The following is a list of 'cool tools' that worked for my children who both have more severe tactile issues:

- *Fidget or awareness box:* I never had a word for this until my daughter began OT, but we always had a little box where she kept her favorite things. I didn't realize at the time that it was filled with things that she liked and that made her hands feel good. She liked smooth little toys that she could rub and she liked the feel of soft material, like fleece. Your fidget/ awareness box should contain objects that give different sorts of sensations such as rough, smooth, furry, sticky, wooly, light, heavy, etc. Ours has different sized Koosh balls, a sponge ball, a squeeze ball, sticky fish, wood with sandpaper glued to it, feathers, a shave brush, toe dividers (used while painting toenails) and various sorts of stretchy guys my kids could squish, stretch and rub. You can purchase complete fidget/ awareness boxes from online sensory stores or you can create your own, having your child pick and choose his favorite things. Just be sure to add in your own choices that fill in the gaps because he may only stick to items that he finds most comfortable.

- *Vibrating Pen:* Vibration is both stimulating and calming for many children with SPD. You can find these in toy stores or at dollar stores. This gadget couples vibration with a favorite fun-time activity (writing or drawing). Other ways to use vibration is with moving stuffed animals, electric tooth-brushes, massage pillows or blankets. As a side note, if your child avoids brushing his teeth, using the vibrating pen with the OT might help him become better about brushing teeth with an electric toothbrush.

- *Weighted vests:* You can find these rather easily now and many are made to look less 'therapeutic' so a child won't feel self-conscious when wearing one. Not only does this help with touch, but it also helps with proprioception, giving children that deep-pressure calming sensation. Other weight products to try include *weighted blankets*, which help with settling down at night for sleep; *lap cozies* which your child can use at school or at home to help with concentration; or *weighted gloves, anklets or sleeves* to be worn during play to get some extra tactile/proprioception. All of these products can be found at most sensory stores, but you can also make them rather easily. For example, we had four different lap cozies with different weights, smells and colors.
Note: Always be sure to keep your child's size and weight in mind when creating or buying a weighted product. Even if they seem to need more weight than other children do, you don't want them to get hurt.

- *Soft pressure brush:* Many children respond well to brushing, but be sure to have your OT or other trained professional teach you the correct brushing method. When done incorrectly, it can cause anxiety.

- *Tactile bars/boards:* We got this idea from an actual sensory store. All you have to do is find different textured materials or substances and stick them to bars or a board. You can mix them all up or have separate bars/boards that have a textural theme (e.g.: soft, rough, fuzzy, etc.) This can be a great addition to your Sensory Game list.

- *Bumpy seat cushion/wedge:* These are seat pads that have a textured and smooth side. They come in a variety of sizes, colors and shapes but the best ones are round or wedge-shaped. These give children tactile input and pressure and also help with fidgeting because your child can squirm around on them without distracting those around her as much.

- *Box of crafts:* We have a shelf full of different tubs of crafty things. Play-Doh, pompoms, feathers, bells, pipe cleaners, glue, sparkles, Moon Sand, different types of fabric, beads and anything else. Crafting is a great way to get your child to experience different sensations.

- *Rice box:* Great for both tactile and proprioceptive input. Have your child decorate a shoebox as she chooses, or purchase a gift box with a lid), fill it with rice or small pasta, then find small toys or fidgets to put into the box. The idea is to get your child to press the toys into the rice/pasta (exertion and pressure) then dig them back up.

- *Seamless clothing:* SOFT Clothing and many other companies offers clothing without tags or seams in them, including underwear. I sure wish these places had been around when my sensory kids were younger. It would have saved so much time and energy cutting tags out of everything. If your child fights getting dressed, avoid a great deal of stress for all involved and purchase, or make, seamless/tagless clothes.

A few years ago, there weren't many games we could play with our kids that didn't cause one of my sensory kids to throw themselves on the floor in frustration after only a few minutes. There are now a variety of options for parents using many of the tools listed above. Here were a few of our favorites:

- *Finger painting options:* Many tactile-sensitive children are reluctant to take part in activities that get their hands dirty, such as finger painting, but they may still really want to try it. Before my daughter was willing to try the shaving cream game (described next), I slowly introduce her to it by getting her used to the sensation of the paint in her hands *without* getting them dirty (by keeping the paint in a sealed plastic bag). After that I introduced a game in which she'd have the *option* of getting them dirty. Put different colored paints in sandwich bags then have your child squish and manipulate the paint through the bags. She will get the idea of how the paint feels, but in a way that isn't threatening to her. From there, you can have her mess around with the paint while wearing gloves or baggies on her hands. Finally, you can have your child play the Food Painting Game. Cook spaghetti or other long pasta, then let it cool off. Have your child 'paint' with the spaghetti by rolling it, slapping it on the paper, dipping it in the paint then throwing/dropping it onto paper or through some other creative way. You can also cut a potato in half then make shapes in the cut side of each half to make stamps. Once my girl was able to do these tasks with little anxiety, I was able to introduce her to the next game.

- *Shaving cream hand painting.* Most days, my daughter avoided activities that got her hands dirty. But after tying this game with Kathy, I incorporated it into her Sensory Diet. Find a place with an easy-to-clean surface, such as the basement floor or a table covered with a vinyl tablecloth. Then squirt out a few piles of the shaving cream and have your child make shapes, faces, play Tic-Tac-Toe or make stories up using shaving cream pictures. If your child seems anxious, be sure to have the sink filled with water or have antiseptic wipes nearby for him to clean his hands with. Alternative products to try include hand/body lotion, hair gel, mousse or dish soap. It's a good idea to start with non-scented versions of these products then, as your child seeks more stimulation, try different scents.

- *Sandbox fun*: I had an outside sandbox that had water table attached to it as well as a small tabletop version that my daughter used on the kitchen table. Each sandbox had different forms of sand. The outside one had coarse, heavy sand whereas the one inside had light, soft sand that felt more like flour. If my daughter needed more tactile stimulation on a particular day, and if she could handle it, we played outside (when the weather was nice) and when her hands didn't feel as happy, we used her tabletop version. It can be used dry or get it wet to make sandcastles and shapes or bury little toys in the sand and dig them back up.

- *Play-Doh movies*: You can use regular Play-Doh for this or try the recipe we shared earlier and scent it up, if he can handle it. Have your child gather a collection of little toys, little people characters, McDonald's prizes or other similar miniature toys. All you do after that is pick or make up movies and use the Play-Doh as props or costumes. My kids could have played this for hours if I'd let them. Have some tools on hand to work with the Play-Doh, such as plastic scissors, rolling pins, cookie cutters and those fancy kitchen gadgets you rarely use like mini juicers, plastic graters, ice cream scoops or even a garlic press.

- *Happy Feet obstacle course*: I set up different versions of obstacle courses at home, patterned from those I learned in sensory integration therapy (you'll learn more about vestibular/proprioceptive exercises in the next chapter). This particular obstacle course is good for touch and pressure. Place different textured items for your child to step on, arranged in a circle. Some suggestions include different types of carpet, a large stuffed animal or 'fur' rug, bubble wrap, one of your tactile boards, cardboard, textured seat cushion/ wedge, lily pads (these are small, round air-filled pads used for balance and coordination), heating or cooling pads, a tray filled with sand, etc. Have your child take his socks and shoes off then venture around the different 'steps'. Make even more fun by creating different ways to move around the course (running, hopping, crawling) or by switching the 'steps' with different items.

- *The Pizza Game*: We touched on this one in earlier chapters. I ended almost every Sensory Diet time with this game. As I've discussed, children with high tactile sensitivities often crave deep pressure and massage. This game is fabulous for that input. All you need is a large ball or yoga ball. Have your child lie down on his Crash Pad (see vestibular exercises in the next chapter) couch cushions on the floor or on a comforter. Start by asking your child what kind of pizza toppings he'd like. Your child is the pizza, so everything goes on him. First, spread the make-believe sauce on him, firmly but gently, rub his body, paying special attention to knees, elbows, fingers, toes and other joints. For each topping, chop, cut, squish or slice all over his torso, arms and legs. When all the toppings are chosen, you need to knead the dough, then ask him how he'd like his crust: light and fluffy or hard and crunchy. His answer tells you how hard he'd like you to roll the ball over his body (most times my daughter asked for a 'super-duper hard crust'). Variations of this game include the Sandwich Game (use sandwich toppings and toast the bread), Hot Dog game (your child is the wiener and you put the toppings on him then roll him up tightly in a comforter or blanket 'bun') or Mexican Food Game (all the toppings with hard, crunchy taco or soft burrito wrap).

- *Cut and paste*: Glue and my sensory kids were not friends, but they did enjoy crafting. So I got a few magazines from my collection, brought down the craft box and had a wonderful time making crafty, touchy/feely pictures. I had glue sticks, glue bottles and liquid glue so they could choose the one they wanted to use. Glue bottles are great for strengthening hands because your child needs to squeeze them. You can also offer the option of putting glue into a container for your child and have him glue with a paint-brush. Be sure to offer different sensations like feathers, pompoms, textured materials and the other things I suggest, including them in your craft box.

- *The Feeling Bucket*: This game has double purpose. It helps your child desensitize himself to certain sensations, and gives him a tool to find meaning in things and how they make him feel. You can do this three different ways, depending on his sensitivity levels and what his body is craving. The first option is to blindfold your child or ask him to close his eyes if he doesn't like the blindfold, and put various objects in his hands. Have a good variety of items with different textures and temperatures like sandpaper (rough), cold spaghetti noodles (slimy/squishy), feathers (soft), flour (fluffy), cotton balls (fuzzy), peeled grapes or pudding (cold/mushy) and ice (cold/hard). Get him to rub each item between his hands, squish, poke or otherwise interact with it then ask him questions like, "What does this feel like?" or "How does it make your hands feel". Or "What's a good describing word or name for that?" The other option is to put things into different containers and have him put his hands into the buckets to manipulate the objects. Then ask the series of questions. The last option is to throw a bunch of different items into a 'Feeling Bucket' and have him pull one of them out. Proceed through the rest of the steps of the game.

There are many other game suggestions but these are the top ones you can use daily. There is always room to change things up as your child's needs, abilities and wants change.

Keep in mind that you can also combine any of the game or exercise suggestions in this chapter to tap into as many of your child's exteroceptors that she can handle at one time. Be sure to watch for sensory overload, and always have her favorite calm-down activity close by.

6

Exercising Your Child's Proprioceptors

In elementary school, you learned all about the *five* senses. Like me, you may have always had a gut feeling that there were other 'senses' but you didn't know the names of them. It wasn't until my daughter began sensory integration therapy that I finally learned the names for those other sensory systems: vestibular and proprioceptive. I also learned that any children with SPD have other sensory-related issues, such as oral-motor (which was covered in Chapter three), motor planning, fine and gross motor skills, bilateral coordination (coordinating both sides of the body) and crossing the body's midline (e.g.: passing a ball from one hand to the other or putting on a jacket).

Once you learn about all of these seven senses, and understand how they are all interrelated, it makes what we're doing with them to make the Sensory Diet more meaningful. This chapter covers activities for balance and movement (vestibular), body awareness (proprioceptive), plus there's a section on activities for motor planning, fine motor skills and helping your child with his bilateral coordination. This chapter concludes by discussing the importance of helping your child's interoceptor system by tapping into her creative side through music, art, writing, poetry, dance and/or reading.

Exercises for the Vestibular System

What I've learned about helping a child move is that once you find a few basic exercises she likes and feels comfortable with, you can expand on those exercises or make up new ones. First, I'd like to discuss the tools and equipment you may find helpful. There's really no need to go out and spend hundreds of dollars on building a sensory gym for your child. Many parents have been able to build the basics on their own or find equipment in the second-hand or Salvation Army-types of stores and then tweak the object to their child's needs.

As you may already know, children with vestibular issues need to crash, spin, jump, bounce, swing, roll, climb, rock, balance, hang and make many other movements. All you really need to do is provide a safe place for your child to do these things. And, if you are able to, also make the following items available to help them with these activities. You can either purchase these items from a sports or sensory store or make them yourself. We made almost all of our own equipment.

- *For crashing:* Pile of pillows, a futon cover filled with foam, gym mats, couch cushions, a blowup pool filled with foam or balls, air mattress or old bed mattress.

- *For spinning:* Go out on the front lawn and spin away (if it's too cold or raining, use the basement or clear a space in a larger room in the house), sitting spin disc, such as Rotation Board, Round-A-Bout, or Playskool Sit 'n Spin Classic (these are discs with a wheel in the middle that the child sits cross-legged around and spins herself around). Or roll down a grassy hill or hop on a merry-go-round at the park.

- *For jumping/bouncing:* Trampoline, skipping rope, couch (if allowed), air mattress, Hippity-Hop ball, yoga ball, pogo sticks (we had one that squeaked every time it was jumped on).

- *For swinging:* Swings (there are many different varieties such as tire, hammock, platform, egg-shaped or seated) or sheets (each end held by caregivers or secured safely to poles). Can be set up inside or outside and can also be used for spinning input.

- *For rocking:* Rocking chair, yoga ball, teeter-totter, T-stool (which is exactly what it sounds like – a stool shaped like a 'T'. You can get one through online sensory stores or you can easily build one yourself), an old baby car seat or textured seat cushions.

- *For balance:* Balance board (can be bought at most sport stores in the yoga section or built by attaching a wooden plank to a circular shaped piece of wood or half of a small yoga ball tailored to the child's size), balance arch (basically a set of wooden rounded monkey bars on the ground), river stones (round, plastic textured steps that can be piled up for varying degrees of difficulty and ability), balance beam, tactile path (a balance beam that is textured and wavy for added coordination practice), stepping stones, step-aerobic board, lily pads (small balance discs) or T-stool.

- *For climbing:* Climbing wall, climbing rope, a rug-covered rope, tree, fence, or ladder. Obviously parental supervision is necessary with climbing activities.

- *For hanging:* Trapeze, acrobatic rings, chin-up bar, monkey bars (jungle gym).

- *For motion (zooming):* Scooter board, ride-on toy, bike, slip-and-slide, skateboard, scooter, toboggan or crazy carpet (in the winter), wagon (in the summer) or slide.

Before I get to our exercise suggestions, there are a couple of important points you should always keep in mind. First, as mentioned in Chapter Three on exercising the exteroceptors, never force your child to do exerting exercises simply because it's exercise time. If his body isn't ready for the activities, or if he needs some other form of stimulation at that time, doing these exercises may hinder rather than help him. Watch his mood, read his needs then decide what would work best. He may need a massage instead of a good bouncy game.

When I first began doing vestibular and proprioceptive exercises at home with my daughter, Kathy advised us to pay close attention to signs of overstimulation or distress from too much input. Just because your sensational child loves the movements doesn't mean you should allow him to go on as long as he wants. As in other areas in their lives, these children don't always recognize when their bodies have had enough stimulation for one session and, in the end, it could actually cause harm. When our kids were in distress and on the verge of a sensory overload meltdown, I could see it on their faces. Their skin color changed, they fidgeted, they rocked and blinked excessively.

Here are other signs that your child may be in distress:

- Avoiding interaction (e.g.: leaning away from you, hugging herself, hiding her face, avoiding eye contact, inappropriate laughing, etc.).

- Rapid breathing or heart rate.

- Crying or close to tears and/or asking to cease activity.

- Moving in a disorganized way (e.g.: falling, unbalanced, flopping down etc.).

- Complaining of stomachache or not feeling well.

- Displaying nervous habits (e.g.: hand flapping, fidgeting, making noises, chewing/picking fingers, etc.).

- Completely shutting down (e.g.: stop speaking, zoning out).

If your child displays any of the above symptoms, or other symptoms that indicate stimulation overload, stop immediately and move to a 'safe' place or calming strategy. Don't be concerned if you have to stop an activity as you can always try again the next day. You're trying to help his body and pushing him too much won't do that.

Keeping these tips in mind, here are some great vestibular exercises we tried:

- *Scooter Board Bowling:* sYou can play this with plastic bowling pins, Tupperware containers, Bottle Buddies (see "Exercises for the Proprioceptive System" later in the chapter on how to make them), paper towel rolls or any other light containers you have on hand. Set up your pins the traditional way or have your child set them up his own way, on a smooth, non-carpeted surface. Have your child lie down on his scooter board on his tummy. Count to three then shoot him gently toward the pins. Give him one point for each pin he knocks down. For more input, you can have him start on a small ramp.

- As an alternative to this game is Scooter Board Tag, which is played with two or more people. Each person has a cloth or rag tucked into the back of his or her pants. All players put their feet up against a wall, chair or some other stable object. Count to three then push off and try to grab someone's cloth. Each cloth grabbed earns the player one point and the person with the most points wins.

- One more alternative is Scooter Board Power Hugs. Two people lie on their scooter boards facing each other then push themselves off of something or use their arms to pull themselves toward each other and hug. If you don't have a scooter board and aren't able to construct one yourself, try Body Bowling instead (see "Exercises for the Proprioceptive System").

- *Bouncy Basketball:* If you don't have a basketball hoop, you can play with a big container, pot, box, old lampshade with the wiring taken out or shoot into the couch or other safe furniture. Have your child bounce on her trampoline (or air mattress or couch cushions) while shooting the ball into the basket at the same time. To challenge her proprioception further, use mini-weighted yoga balls and/or have her slam dunk the ball. We use a variety of different size balls, give a shot maximum (usually three) and keep score. Having rules and boundaries helps keep your child focused and organized.

- *T-Stool Fishing:* The fishing game I described earlier can be used with the T-stool as well to help your child with balance. The point of this game is to have your child work on his balance and help his body learn to hold a steady position. If he seems a little uncertain about the feel of the T-stool at first, allow him to ease into it by either leaning it up against a wall so he can practice or using a yoga ball. Other alternatives to fishing are doing songs with motions, such as "Johnny Works With One Hammer", "Hot Potato", "Hokey Pokey" or any other of his favorites. These songs challenge your child to hold his balance as he lifts legs, moves arms and jiggles around.

- *Steady Freddy Coconut Toss:* Earlier, I described how to create your own coconut tree with a Bobo doll. This is a game you can play with that tree. Have your child balance on her balance board. If you don't have one, you can place a longer board perpendicularly on top of a narrower piece of wood so it resembles a mini seesaw. Have your child toss the coconuts at the tree and try to get all of them to stick. For an added challenge, you can shake the tree (mimicking an earthquake) while she's tossing the coconuts.

- *[Your child's name]'s Awesome Obstacle Course:* This was one of my daughter's favorite games to play with Kathy. The best part is that you can work with your child to create the best obstacle course for him. It's a personalized combination of his favorite activities, along with a few that he may normally avoid, just to make sure he gets a complete vestibular and proprioceptive workout. Usually what I did for my kids was combine activities for upper body strength (e.g.: Body Bowling), squeezing (crawling through a tunnel or other tight space), jumping, heavy lifting/ carrying/ throwing of an object, climbing then end with crashing. This combination gives your child's body everything it needs to feel more organized. The activities you choose to put together with your child can be from your OT's recommendations or things that you've tweaked on your own.

- *Animal Dice:* This is a game that can help your child with vestibular input while also providing an activity that the whole family can have fun with. The only things you need are poster board paper (any color), pictures of animals (either Word ClipArt or pictures from magazines) and your own imagination. Mark the poster board into the outer surfaces so it can fold into a cube[1]. Cut it out and tape or staple it together securely. Then choose six different animals for your dice. Pick animals that are both familiar and have great moves, like a snake, horse and/or monkey. Give each person a chance to roll. Whatever animal shows up, the roller has to imitate. Everyone in our house had tons of fun with this game. You can create different dice with animals that make particularly noisy sounds or that make funkier moves or a combination.

- *Towel Roll Baseball:* Or course there's nothing wrong with getting out there and playing a 'real' game of baseball, but this is a great safe inside alternative as well as a great way to start teaching your child the body coordination involved with playing the actual game. All you need for this game are empty paper towel rolls and a few blown-up balloons. Decide where the bases will be, then choose one person to be the pitcher and another to bat first. The pitcher either tosses or bobs the balloon with his bat to the batter, who tries to hit it. This is a hilarious game that gets your child moving and learning about teamwork, sequential steps in play and other important skills. This can also be the base for other team sports like volleyball or tennis.

  Tip: For added stimulation, have the batter lie down or sit on a swing while trying to hit the balloon.

---

[1] http://printables.atozteacherstuff.com/435/cube-pattern/ or simply Google "cube template". ULINE.com has pre-cut "cube boxes" from 3" to 20" square.

- *Pool Noodle Soccer:* Blow up a balloon. Choose two different sides for the soccer goals, then use a pool noodle, which provides extra vestibular input as your child tries to coordinate the noodle, to get the balloon into the other person's goal. If you don't have a pool noodle, you can also use a paper towel roll, if it isn't demolished after the baseball game described above.

- *Bopping to Tunes:* This can be played with either a Bobo doll, an actual punching bag from a toy or sports store or you can create a type of punching bag yourself. All you need is a body pillowcase filled with newspaper, shopping bags or other forms of stuffing. Tie the bag closed and hang it from the ceiling. Find your child's favorite music track and have her punch away in time to the music or sing your own songs while bopping away. This can also be used as part of your child's Awesome Obstacle Course.

- *Hippity-Hop Hide-and-Seek:* Ask your child to cover her eyes while you hide various stuffed animals or other toys around the room. Be sure to limit the hiding and seeking to a specific area so it doesn't become too overwhelming for your child. Place objects in relatively easy-to-find places or at least in places your child can find with a few hints. Once everything is hidden, have your child search for the objects. You can give the hot and cold hints when she is close to an object and offer hints when she runs into trouble. As she finds each toy, have her bounce on her hippity-hop ball with the toy in hand, back over to a box or crash place. This game is great for gravity, balance, visual discrimination and core body strength.

- *Swing Bumps:* This is a great vestibular and proprioceptive game, if you have room for two swings in your sensory space, that's great. Otherwise you can always play this at the park or another place with two swings next to each other. Tire swings are the ideal type of swing for this game. Both players sit in their swings so that they are facing each other. Then both people swing toward the other, trying to bounce the other off her swing. The caution for this game is that a child with higher vestibular or tactile needs may bump harder than the other player does, so it's important to set some rules and boundaries in place from the start. Of course, you would only do this outdoors in a setting with a padded landing area or air mattresses under the swing.

Take the activity ideas shared above and make them your own by changing tools, equipment or even the rules of how you play the game. Later in the chapter, we'll detail a few exercises and games that can help a child who has problems with crossing the midline and bilateral coordination.

Exercises for the Proprioceptive System

The main thing to remember about your child's proprioceptive system is that you're trying to connect the neural pathways that allow him to understand what his muscles and joints are supposed to be doing. I always knew when my daughter needed extra proprioceptive input because she'd walk around on her tiptoes and tripped and fell more than usual. Your goal is to strengthen your child's muscles while giving her the heavy input her joints need.

Children with proprioceptive issues need to pull, push, lift, drag, hang, carry, stretch and squeeze. Here are a few sensory tools and ideas for the proprioceptive system:

- *For pulling:* Pull toys, wagon/sled or scooter board carrying a friend or sibling or small load of objects, Dad's tool belt or yoga resistance bands.

- *For pushing:* Swing, wall push-ups, chair push-ups, shopping cart, push toys, wheelbarrow, sandbox (similar to using the Rice Box where you have your child push small objects into the sand and dig them up or even wet the sand for extra weight).

- *For lifting:* Milk jugs, mini-weighted yoga balls, Bottle Buddies (see how to make your own later in this chapter), stuffie buddies (weight-stuffed animals, beanbags or other items) or helping to carry/unload groceries.

- *For pressure:* Weighted vest, lap cozies, weighted blankets, wheelbarrow walks (child is on his hands and knees, parent stands behind him and pull his legs up so he's supporting himself with his hands then the child walks around like he's a wheelbarrow) and vibrating toys or tools.

- *For dragging:* Suitcase/backpack on wheels, pillowcase full of balls or blocks, a jump rope or pool noodle with something heavy tied to one end.

- *For hanging:* Trapeze, acrobatic rings, monkey bars or gym rope.

- *For carrying:* Full backpack, fanny pack, full milk jugs or grocery bags.

- *For stretching:* Yoga or Brain Dance.

- *For squeezing:* Stress balls, tent tunnels, wrapping up in a blanket, squeezing between two chairs/furniture and wall/etc., Body Sox (full-body Lycra socks available through online sensory stores) and deep pressure massage.

These were the form of exercises and play that my kids always avoided. I didn't notice at first because they were always running, spinning, jumping and crashing. It wasn't until they started SI therapy that I was told that, my daughter especially, had a very strong lower body but that her upper body was quite weak (e.g.: she struggled sitting up from lying down, holding or throwing heavy things, or pulling herself up on a trapeze or climbing wall). I simply began to incorporate one or two of the following exercises into her regular Sensory Diet session and another one or two throughout her day.

As with any of these exercises, only do what your child is able to cope with, encourage her to try even if she feels like she can't do it and reward her with her favorite calm-down activity when she's done.

Here are a few great exercises and activities to help the proprioceptive system:

- *Horsey Carriage:* If you have a wagon, have your child pretend to be the horsey for a carriage ride, pulling either a smaller sibling or an object with some weight, keeping your child's strength and size in mind. If you don't have a wagon (or toboggan in the winter), have your child pull heavy objects or a smaller child around on the floor in a sheet or blanket. To make it more fun, you can sing songs, do fancy footsteps or have a race.

- *Bottle Buddy Body Bowling:* Try saying *that* 10 times! Your pins in this game can be regular pins, paper towel rolls, empty containers or full cans for extra weight. Doing it with Bottle Buddies is much more fun. Make your own using a few empty pop or juice bottles, colorful sparkles, confetti, sprinkles, food coloring and some duct tape. Of course, you would never use glass bottles—only plastic. Put a few spoonfuls of each of your goodies in the bottle first. If the lip of your bottle is too small, you can use a funnel to get everything inside. Then fill the bottle up to just below the neck with water. Add a few drops of food coloring, if you choose to, screw the cap on as tightly as possible then wrap a few layers of duct tape around it for added security.

• To play the game, line up your Bottle Buddies, bowling pins or a combination of both. Have your child move a few feet away from the pins then wheelbarrow walk him down to knock the pins over with his arms. For an added challenge, have him move back a little further away from the pins with each try. Do it a few times until his arms feel tired, but he's not exhausted.

• *Pool Noodle Rolls:* A shorter, fatter version of the pool noodle is required for this exercise or you can also use cylinder-shaped pillows or cushions. Have your child lie down on her tummy. Take two of the noodles or cushions, placing one under your child's thighs and the other under her tummy. Have your child stretch her arms out in front of her, this is the starting position. Then ask her to pull her body forward with her palms, similar to the movement the hands and arms make when crawling, until she's doing almost a Cobra Pose, as in yoga (arms pushing her up but her lower body still lying flat on the noodles or cushion), then have her push herself slowly back to the original position. This helps to exercise her upper body. Be sure she breathes in as she pulls up, then breathes out as she pushes herself back. This exercise can be extremely calming and helps get your child in tune with her body.

• *Laundry Basket Races:* Have a laundry basket or box for each racer. Fill each racer's basket/box with items like phone books, cans, bags of dried beans, bottled water or heavier toys. Have the racers line up on one side of the room (or yard, if you're playing outside). Count down from three, then yell, "Go!" The first person to push his basket/box to the other side and back again wins. Be sure that your child doesn't try zooming so fast to win that he topples over the basket. He should go fast enough to keep going, but not so fast to get hurt. You can also do the same game *pulling* the basket/box. Have your child use his hands or tie a rope on the basket/box to make it easier.

- *Body Sox Antics:* We were introduced to the Body Sox during my daughter's SI therapy program. Body Sox are fabulous for helping with body awareness and they also offer hugging-like pressure and resistance. Before doing any fun games with the sock, however, have your child get into it with her head sticking out of it. As calming as the sock can be for most children, it can also be distressing for others who have tactile, vestibular and proprioception issues. Once he feels safe with it, see if he's willing to pull himself completely inside of it. Then try getting him to:

  - Stretch out like a star.

  - Roll, squirm or slither like an inchworm or snake.

  - Bump into things set up for him and have him guess what they are (be sure to supervise your child closely for this one).

  - Play the Caterpillar Game—Have him pretend he's a caterpillar getting ready to change into a butterfly. He can squirm around to his swing or crash place then pop his head out of the opening of his sock. Finally, he stretches his arms out and flutters like a butterfly.

- *Can I Take Your Order?* We made this game up after watching my son trying to carry a tray filled with his toy cars from his car shelf to the coffee table. Then he came over to me, handed me a car and gestured for me to eat it. We had a whole box full of pretend food, but you don't need to have real-looking food to play this game. Your child can use canned goods, bags of beans or cereal or, like my son did, use his favorite little toys. Whatever you decide to use, make sure it has a bit of weight to it. The 'waiter' comes over, takes your order then goes back to the 'kitchen' to get the food. When he brings it back, he can carry it with both hands in front of him, try to balance it on his shoulders or head or even drag it, if it's a heavier order. An add-on for this game is to have one person in the 'kitchen' cooking the food with pots, pans or bakeware before passing it along to the 'waiter'. This game helps with following steps in an activity, balance, coordination and body awareness.

- *Fun With Boxes:* When my daughter was very small, she loved squishing herself into small boxes or crawling through small spaces. Until I learned more about SPD and the needs of the proprioceptive system, I didn't realize she'd been doing that in order to feel things. All children seem to like boxes, often they like the box than whatever was inside the box in the first place. I actually had a collection of boxes of various sizes in our basement in case we ever wanted to mail things, create things or just to have fun with. One of my daughter's favorite things to do was to see how small a box she could squish herself into before she felt that she was too big. Other times, she liked to throw stuffed animals into a larger box then get right in there with it. We even had a large box from which we cut out windows and a door. The kids all helped decorate it with stickers, markers, crayons and paint.

- *Chair Tug-Of-War*: This great old-fashioned game is good for your child's joints, muscles, hand strength and bilateral coordination. Use a thick rope, towel, sheet or jump rope. Your child and either a sibling or friend sit in chairs facing each other a few feet apart. Their feet need to be flat on the floor. Each person takes one end of the rope and the first person to pull the other off his chair wins. Make sure that your child has a strong enough grip in order to pull and be pulled. The skill will strengthen the more he plays but it may be frustrating at first for a child whose hand grip is weaker. This can also be a great rough play activity for times when your child may not be comfortable with actual touch.

- *Blueberry and Raspberry Relay Race*: This helps with motor-planning, body awareness, movement and toning muscles. We had a red two-pound yoga ball (raspberry) and a blue five-pound one (blueberry). If you don't have yoga balls, you can play the game with bags of dried beans or canned goods. Set up one item on one side of the room and your second, heavier item on the other side. When you say, "Go!" your child rushes to pick up the first item, run it to the second one, exchange them, then run back with the heavier item. Give him a crash mat to jump into after reaching the starting point again. This is a more advanced game in which a child can basically follow the instructions and not get too 'lost'. If he appears to struggle, simplify the game by having him run over to the first object only, bring it back, then crash. A second game can be set up with the heavier object.

- *Hula Hoop Dancing*: This is a great game for body awareness. For extra auditory input, you can put steel or regular marbles in the hula hoop so it makes a cool noise when your child spins it. This is a simple but fun game. All you have to do is put on her favorite CD and spin away. If your child has trouble with moving her hips to get the hoop to go, just have her use her arms, legs or even neck, if she can. Have her lie down and just roll with the hoop or have her throw it so that it rolls away from her and she can chase it. Use your imagination and expand on the game as your child's abilities increase.

Activities for Fine Motor Skills

These are only a few examples of games and activities. Feel free to change them to suit your child's abilities, sensitivities and preferences. As promised, these are a few suggestions for fine motor skills, bilateral coordination and motor planning.

- Beading.
- Scrapbooking.
- Cut-and-paste.
- Counting coins/putting them into a piggy bank.
- Sorting games, like with cards.
- Lite-Brite.
- Puzzles.
- Mosaic art crafts.
- Coloring, writing and drawing.
- Water games using eyedroppers or squirt guns.

- Play-Doh using a cutting knife or plastic scissors.

Activities for Motor Planning

Kids with motor planning difficulties struggle with instructions or knowing when and how to start/stop activities. These are great games that help teach them about directions, instructions and walking them through the steps. If you notice your child struggling with any activity, do it with him, guiding his movements so he feels how his body is supposed to go, and give him some ankle/wrist/glove weights to help give him feedback on what his body is doing. Ask him questions so the thinks things through, offer hints, give him visual cues or have him write things down on a dry-erase board or chalkboard, whatever helps him 'get' the steps and retain them.

- Animal walks (try the Animal Dice game), getting the child to move in different directions like forward, backward, sideways, etc.

- Hopscotch.

- [Your child's name], the Treasure Hunter. Create a map with step-by-step directions to get to the 'X' at the end.

- Games like Simon Says, Mother May I, What Time Is It Mr. Wolf or The Mirror Game (child mirrors your movements).

- Obstacle Course with hurdles the child has to get around, through or over. Have him talk through how to solve the problem in order to go on.

- Sports games like baseball, basketball, floor/ice hockey, relay races in which he has to maneuver around objects, etc.

Activities for Bilateral Coordination

As discussed in Chapter Five, bilateral coordination is the ability to move both sides of our bodies in a coordinated way *together* or using the two sides of the body for different things (e.g.: throwing a ball in the air with one hand and whacking it with a tennis racket with the other). It means being able to pass something from one hand to the other or understanding how to move the feet, one in front of the other, to walk, climb stairs or jump. Some children need help with making the connections to do these tasks, and the following activities can help:

- Music-and-motion songs such as, 'Head, Shoulders, Knees and Toes' or the sorts of songs The Wiggles sang.

- Big movement activities requiring the legs and arms to work together to accomplish an end goal like cartwheels, jumping rope, dancing, yoga, aerobics or jumping jacks.

- Tip: At our local sports store, where I got a lot of the sensory equipment we used, I picked up a set of foam dice that have numbers on one die (2, 4, 6, 8, 10, 12) and movements (toe touches, jumping jacks, push-ups, sit ups, hop on one foot, arm circles) on the other. The idea is to roll both dice together to get the type of movement and how many must be done. Some children may not like this one at first but it's a great family game and helps to wake up a tired body. Also, you don't have to pay the $12 at the store as you can make your own version using poster paper (just like Animal Dice).

- Tai Chi, Taekwondo, Karate, Jiu Jitsu and similar activities help coordinate the body as well as get your child more in tune with his body and how it moves. It also helps to increase self-esteem because your child earns colored belts as his skills increase.

Activities for Helping with
Crossing the Midline and/or Bilateral Coordination

Carol Kranowitz describes the ability to cross the midline as, "...using the eye, hand or foot of one side of the body in the space of the other eye, hand or foot." So, for example, a child who has difficulty in this area would color on the right side of a coloring book with her right hand and on the left side with her left hand. Or she would draw a horizontal line with her right hand then switch to her left when she gets to her midline to finish the line. It's almost like there is no connection that the motion or movement is continuous or that the body works *together* to complete such tasks effectively.

These are a few ideas to help work on this problem and strengthen midline skills:

- Hand-and-Motion songs like 'Head, Shoulders, Knees and Toes', most songs by The Wiggles (e.g.: Monkey Dance, Here Comes the Bear, Wags the Dog, etc.) or any song that requires your child to use both sides of his body with repetitive actions in different ways.

- Have your child help with baking or cooking by opening jars and containers, getting stuff out of the fridge, measuring out and dumping ingredients into the bowl and stirring. This is also great for gross motor skills, eye-hand coordination and using tools.

- Play 'Follow the Leader' (we used to call it 'Mirror Mama' or Mirror [your child's name]'). This great game teaches your child about body awareness and crossing the midline. Be sure to move slowly and do a lot of moves that involve moving one side of the body across the other, such as one hand on the opposite shoulder, crossing one foot over the other or twisting from one side to the other.

- Games like 'Hot Potato' are excellent for midline skills, since you're taking the potato from one side of you and passing it to the other side (without transferring the potato to the other hand). Try playing the game to music so you can go faster or slower to the beat and even change direction.

- Set up a paint easel, spread paper across the floor or hang paper on the outside of the house or on a fence. Then have your child paint pictures of objects he sees that make him move left and right and up and down. You can also do this with sidewalk chalk.

- Swimming is an excellent activity for bilateral coordination because your child needs to use his hands, arms, legs and feet *together* in order to stay afloat or move. Swimming instructors not only teach how to move the arms and legs, but also different ways of moving the body, breath control, visual skills and more. If you have access to a facility like the YMCA, many of the instructors have experience with helping children with developmental and other issues.

- Yoga, as I mentioned earlier, is a fantastic form of exercise to help with calming, stretching the muscles and bilateral coordination.

- Gymnastics, especially tumbling, balancing, ribbon and rhythm forms are especially good for proprioception and bilateral coordination.

Difficulties in the vestibular and proprioception systems aren't always as obvious as difficulties in other systems because when a child with SPD feels he can't do something, he avoids the activity all together. For example, I didn't realize until she worked with Kathy that my daughter had such serious struggles with things like balance, coordination or bilateral coordination because she avoided all games or activities involving such skills. And I never pushed her to do them because I just wanted her to have fun.

Once you are aware of struggles in these areas, encourage your child to try as many of these activities as you can as a part of her Sensory Diet. At the very least, she won't be fearful of the activities anymore and will be more willing to try new things. And that's our greatest hope: *trying*.

Tuning Into, and Calming Down, the Interoceptors

As explained earlier, most of what goes on in the interoceptor system is beyond our conscious awareness. It involves functions such as our heart rate, breathing, digestion and other bodily functions. Most books about SPD don't discuss this system because it is very complicated and that's also why I only touch on the basics of it in this book. I believe this system is just as important as all the others because it is affected when we are anxious or stressed and your child is very often in that state when his body isn't in sync.

The most important thing you can do to help your child with his interoceptors is to help him feel what's happening to his body when he is in distress.

- Help her connect her internal response to the outer trigger by finding the right words to describe the reactions. "Your eyes are wide and you're chewing your lip. You seem nervous." Putting her response into words helps your child realize, "Yes, that's how I feel."

- Put his hand on his heart and say something like, "Can you feel how fast your heart is beating? We need to slow down a little bit." Then talk about what is making him feel nervous, scared or upset that is causing his heart to beat faster.

- Help him figure out what caused his internal response by using a descriptive word for his feeling. "We were just playing with crayons and I suggested painting. Did my talking about painting make you feel *nervous*? Let's try figuring out why painting makes you *nervous*."

- Have her brainstorm with you on strategies that give her a bit of control over the situation.

Of course, you have to be very in tune with what calms your child and what gets him going because those can be very different for each child. Finger painting, for example, can be just the right messy, fun play for a child who calms with tactile stimulation, whereas the same activity would push a tactile-defensive child over the edge.

Once my daughter got to the point where she could at the very least verbalize what's happening inside her body, we were able to find the right words to describe the feelings and why they were happening so we could figure out together what to do next. Knowing how the body *feels* (the rapid heartbeat, fast breathing, goosebumps, etc.) but not understanding *why*, can increase the stress level as well as sensory symptoms even further.

I found that the most effective activities are those that involve increasing body awareness through the mind-body connection. Many of these therapies are more suitable for older children who are better able to verbalize and follow directions.

Here are a few suggestions:

- *Yoga:* The idea of yoga is to connect the body, mind and spirit. A regular practice of yoga is supposed to help guide us to a sense of peace and well-being as well as instill a feeling of being in tune with our environment. Slowly moving the body into different poses and really concentrating on slow, deliberate breathing is a great way to help our kids become more in tune with their bodies. It is also good for strength, balance, coordination and body awareness. This makes it one of the best-suited additions to our sensational kids overall Sensory Diet.

- *Biofeedback:* As previously discussed, the nervous system is divided into two major parts: voluntary and involuntary. You can control how fast or slowly you breathe, but if you try holding your breath for too long your body will scream, "Air! I need air!" and force you to breathe. A biofeedback therapist helps teach people how to control many of those involuntary functions. The therapist attaches a person to an electroencephalogram (EEG), which monitors the individual's brain activity through electrodes on the scalp. As the patient listens to various tones or visuals, the therapist takes note when a particular trigger causes the EEG to show high levels of activity. She then instructs the person how to relax the body. The point of this process is to teach how certain stimuli affects the body then teaches ways to calm the body back down.

- *Guided Imagery:* This technique doesn't involve any sort of monitoring. It relies on the power of suggestion and helps to reduce anxiety and stress, improve moods and helps to ease pain. The idea is to focus on something so intently that the individual convinces his subconscious that it's real. When you think about it, our sensational kids do this when they tell themselves that something is scary or feels bad. Guided imagery helps the child focus on something else so that scary thing isn't so scary. It's called *guided* because the facilitator is telling a calming story which provides visual cues through verbalization. This can be done live or with an audiobook. One technique Kathy got my daughter to use was picturing a superhero shrinking something that scared her to a tiny size that she could simply blow away. Guided imagery isn't a tactic a lot of people believe in but the power of the mind is strong and just as we can convince ourselves that "we can't", we can also convince ourselves that "we can".

- *Meditation:* Now this doesn't mean you have to get your child to shave her head, dress in a toga and chant to herself into a semi-conscious state as so many seem to believe about meditation. The goal of meditation is to get rid of all the negative thoughts in your head and focus on nothing but slowing down the body and mind. And whether it's lying down while listening to quiet music or sitting still with eyes closed, it's quiet time. Of course, this practice would be very difficult for a child who constantly needs to be on the go, but learning to be still at times is very important. At one point, I got my daughter to write or talk out things on her mind (e.g.: drawing pictures or keeping a 'Feelings Journal') then have her lie down and count to fifty. We often did this at night when she either couldn't get to sleep or woke up and couldn't go back to sleep. In true meditation, one is supposed to focus on a 'mantra' which is a phrase or word that the person repeats while meditating. It's basically a focus trigger.

The whole point is to have your child focus on something other than the stimulus or irritation and bring her body down to a calmer state.

7

Feeding the Hungry Brain

One of the most intense areas of concerns for caregivers of children with SPD is eating. When gustatory, olfactory and, especially, tactile systems are very sensitive, eating can be a huge hurdle. The concern is that these children often aren't getting enough of the vitamins, minerals and essential fatty acids their bodies need to function properly. Because when your child's already hungry brain is starved of these nutritional elements, it can increase her sensory sensitivities.

By the time my daughter turned two, what she ate had dwindled down to just plain pasta, applesauce, macaroni with cheese, milk, and chicken nuggets. This is hardly the diet of champions. It was no wonder, then, that she had trouble keeping weight on, was cranky, ran out of energy quickly and had skin problems. As Kelly Dorfman points out in her Foreword of this book, nutrition and brain function are very closely linked. If the hungry brain isn't getting what it needs, it can't properly communicate with the rest of the body. For children with SPD, this is a serious issue.

Think of what you feel like when you have skipped breakfast or are late eating a meal. You probably feel tired, your stomach hurts, your muscles may feel weak, you may not have enough energy to carry out basic tasks, you might have difficulty concentrating and/or you might be super cranky. Hey! That probably sounds a lot like how your little one behaves. In addition to all of these normal reactions, your child's sensitivity levels may also be higher and her reactions to her environment even more intense than usual.

At this point you are probably asking yourself questions such as: I understand the nutrition guidelines, but what are the most important vitamins, minerals or other nutrients essential to my sensational child's needs? What are possible reasons for my child's eating issues, aside from her sensory issues? How can I get my child to eat the foods she needs when even just talking about certain foods starts her gagging? Is there a way to sneak the foods into her diet without her knowing about it? What other options do I have for getting the nutrients into my child if he's absolutely refusing to eat the foods?

These are some of the most common questions and concerns and this chapter addresses them all and offers a few pearls of wisdom from Kelly Dorfman, M.S., L.D.N, Jane Hersey from Feingold Association and Dana Laake, a nutritionist, dietician and author of *Kid Friendly ADHD & Autism Cookbook*.

Why Won't My Child Eat?

At this point, it's important to discuss possible reasons behind your sensitive child's reluctance to eat. Understanding some of these issues is necessary so that you can take a more holistic approach to encouraging him to eat better.

Common reasons for poor eating include:

- *Sensory systems interfering with eating:* Eating is truly a multi-sensory stimulating experience. We often make our minds up about food based on what it looks like and how it smells, even before we allow that food anywhere near our mouth. A child with high sensitivity levels may even gag just at the sight of a certain food. This is often because a food reminds him of something else he finds unappealing. Try investigating his reactions. Also, if that food gets a stamp of approval for appearance or smell, the child may still reject its texture.

- In addition, a child who struggles with proprioceptive issues may not have the jaw strength to chew properly. Or his tongue may work against him not allowing him to move the food around in his mouth or even to swallow. He may not even be able to tell when his mouth is full, resulting in him spitting the food out, or throwing up anything he's already managed to get down.

- The exercises you're doing with him help with these issues, and there are other tactics you can try at the dinner table to help him work through textures (See tips under 'How Can I Get My Child to Eat' later in this chapter).

- *The tummy's mixed signals:* A child with severe sensory issues isn't always able to tell when he's hungry or if he's had enough to eat. The signals that tell his brain whether or not his tummy is full aren't getting through and he's more likely than other children to associate hunger pains with 'bad' feelings. My son still isn't able to tell when he's had enough to eat and I actually have to say, "I think you've had enough for now." Those 'bad' feelings associated with eating, in addition to the smell, tastes and textures of food, can be enough to turn an overly sensitive child off of eating. Help him to tune into what his tummy needs by talking through what a good portion size is, getting him to describe how his tummy feels *before* he eats then again *after* he's eaten and/or having him sit a few minutes after eating before he gets seconds.

- *Making the dinner table a battleground*: Most parents remember hearing the words, "You'll sit there until you've eaten everything on your plate!" at some point in their child-hood. The problem with statements like this is that it can make mealtime and eating an extremely negative experience for all involved and, honestly, such statements just don't work for a child with high sensitivities. She isn't refusing to eat something to be rebellious or naughty. Often the problem is that she's associated a 'bad feeling' with the food on her plate. Yelling at her or threatening her only intensifies those negative feelings. Instead of making the dinner table a battleground, try finding peaceful ways to ease her into trying foods (see "How Can I Get My Child to Eat?" later in this chapter for tips to get your child interested in trying her food).

- *Connecting eating with eliminating*: Often a child with high tactile defensiveness has trouble with eating *and* eliminating. My daughter hated the feeling of elimination so much that she held it for days. For health reasons, I often had to force her to sit until she released it. Her first OT tried to help ease the anxiety about elimination by reading her a book about pooping, describing in full detail how what we eat ends up coming back out. Once my daughter made the connection between eating and eliminating, it became even more difficult to get her to do either. This is a very tricky situation that is frustrating, worrisome and difficult to change. The best things to do here is keep talking her through it, showing her that her mom, dad and brother/sister *all* eat and poop and get her to connect to the fact that holding it in feels worse than just letting everything come out. Most importantly, teach her that eating isn't what makes the discomfort of pooping happen. *Holding* it does.

- *Having a leaky gut*: This condition isn't a direct result of sensory issues, but the pain and/or discomfort it can cause may contribute to eating problems. The lining of the digestive tract helps to filter out the harmful or unneeded debris in our food, including undigested pieces, while allowing the nutrients and fuel to be absorbed into our bodies. When this lining isn't working properly, the debris that would normally be filtered out leaks into the system, causing an array of developmental, neurological and behavioral problems. And the gas, bloating, loose stools and food intolerances (meaning that certain foods may make the condition worse) cause discomfort that your child associates with food and eating. A nutritionist, dietician or naturopath would be able to diagnose this condition properly and it is possible to repair the gut through an elimination and replacement process (see sidebar "Help For 'Leaky Gut' at the end of the chapter).

What's My Child's Brain Hungry For?

Because SPD is a neurological disorder, it's important to make sure these children get a lot of healthy brain food, including the good omega fats. All children need healthy brain foods, but it's essential for children with SPD for three important reasons:

- The brain is made up of around 60-percent fat, so that means that what we eat literally becomes our brain. If your child isn't getting the right kinds of healthy fat, her brain will make her get it any way she can and she'll turn to the unhealthy saturated fats. The brain craves fat, so learning what the essential brain-friendly fats are will help you choose the foods she needs and, hopefully, get her cravings up for those good fats instead.

- As I've discussed, children with SPD have a tendency to avoid many foods due to their high sensitivity to smells and textures. This can lead to a deficiency in crucial vitamins and minerals that their brains need in order to cope with their symptoms. Learning how to sneak those brain foods into their fussy diets is essential.

- Nutritionists who specialize in SPD and sensory sensitive children have discussed how making simple but important changes to the diet can dramatically reduce sensory symptoms.

Experts say that children will never starve themselves. They always find something they're willing to eat because the discomforts of being really hungry win out. But if you allow your child to always eat plain pasta or chicken nuggets, she isn't going to get all of the essential nutrients her body needs. Plus, remember, your child needs to be exposed to those different smells, tastes and textures in order to create a neural connection for those sensations. And how else is she supposed to understand whether she truly doesn't like a specific food or if it's just the feel she doesn't like?

Research through the Autism Association has shown that children with neurological disorders, such as SPD or autism spectrum disorder, are more vulnerable to becoming 'junk food junkies' by the very nature of their disorders. The neural connection that helps their brains absorb and maintain the 'right' fats it needs isn't there. And, as mentioned, when they don't eat the 'right' fats, their brains take fat in any form it can. I can tell you from experience that my kids would have rather gulped down a greasy hot dog than a muffin packed with flaxseed oil. But, as you'll find out later, it's all about choosing the best forms of the foods they prefer, or tweaking them, then introducing them to other foods by branching out from what they're already comfortable with.

The following is a list of some very important foods to include in your child's diet and reasons to include the food:

- *Tomatoes:* They contain lycopene, one of the strongest carotenoids, which acts as an antioxidant.

- *Figs:* A good source of potassium and fiber, both of which have been shown to improve cognition, as well as vitamin B_6, which is responsible for producing mood-boosting serotonin, lowering cholesterol and preventing water retention.
  Tip: Fig cookies have at least one gram of fiber per cookie. These are yummy, and if you make them yourself, a healthy way to get those figs into your little eater.

- *Broccoli:* Broccoli is considered a 'miracle veggie'. It contains indole-3-carbinol and sulforaphane, lots of vitamin C and beta-carotene.

Tip: Steam it lightly in the microwave or on the stovetop to preserve the phytonutrients. Or, if your sensitive little one likes the crunchier sensation, serve it raw with some homemade dip.

- *Bok choy:* This power veggie contains natural detoxifiers and loads of calcium.

- *Squash:* Winter squash has huge amounts of vitamin and beta-carotene and loads of fiber. And you may get your sensitive child to eat these more easily because most varieties are on the sweeter side. Try slipping them into soups or stews, either in soft chunks or blended in completely.

- *Beans:* They contain B vitamins, slow (complex) carbo-hydrates and plenty of fiber.

- *Milk:* This contains riboflavin (vitamin B_2), important for good vision and good source of vitamin A, which is known to help improve eczema and allergies. Plus, you get tons of calcium and vitamin D too. Tip: If your child is used to higher-fat milk, don't go cold turkey. Instead, mix the two together at first. Or use it to make your favorite smoothie or a cup of hot chocolate. Soy milk is a fantastic alternative if your child has dairy intolerances. Consult your nutritionist before giving skim or 2% milk to children under age 3.

- *Oily fish:* This is probably the single most important element required for optimal brain health. Increased omega-3 intake has been shown to help ease the symptoms of many mental health concerns, including anxiety and irritability as well as your child's SPD symptoms. Fish like wild Alaskan salmon, mackerel and tuna all contain DHA (decosahexaenoic acid), the best form of omega-3.

- *Shellfish:* Contains loads of vitamin B_{12} to help support nerve and brain function, plus iron and hard-to-get minerals like magnesium and potassium.

A few of these foods may be difficult to get into your sensitive child, especially the fish and veggies. In our house, we also have a severe peanut allergy so we have to be careful how we cook things. I also did the research and found other foods that provide the same goodness found in fish as the kids got used to the whole fishy idea.

The following items are considered by leading nutritionists and dieticians to be the top ten brain foods that help enhance brain chemistry, memory, mood and cognition, all of which are so important for your sensational child's optimal brain functions:

- *Eggs:* Eggs contain choline, one of the superstar brain nutrients. Your brain needs choline in order to produce acetylcholine, which plays a critical role in memory.
  Tip: Eggs are one of those tactile sensitive foods that your children with sensory sensitivities often can't deal with. Just remember that eggs can be prepared in several different ways (e.g.: boiled, fried, scrambled or even in a sandwich), so try experimenting with them until something clicks.

- *'Smart' oils:* Olive, walnut, avocado and flax oils are far superior to canola, corn and soy oils, which contain omega-6 fats rather than the preferred omega-3s. Cook, fry or even make your dressings and dips with these rich oils instead.

- *Tempeh:* This isn't the most attractive food, but it's considered a smart protein that helps stabilize blood sugar. Similar to tofu in that it is also made from soybeans, it's fermented which gives your child an extra health boost. This is a great alternative to meat because of its high protein content. Also, because it has no real flavor of its own, you can put it in stir-fry, desserts or even smoothies and it will take on the flavors of what it's cooked with.

- *Flaxseeds:* These are a true super food. Use them sparingly until you adjust to the taste. Flaxseeds are literally made of nothing but fiber, vitamins and omega-3s. They are a must for vegetarians. I mix them in with granola, homemade granola bars, oatmeal and smoothies.

- *Greek yogurt:* Yogurt, the really thick, luscious, fattening kind, contains tyrosine, which perks you up and improves mental alertness. But avoid giving your child too much of the sugary kinds of yogurts. Even better, sweeten the plain stuff yourself with fresh fruit, cinnamon or granola.

- *Raw vegetables:* These are full of fiber, vitamins (especially C and E) and antioxidants. The greener the better but those yellow, orange and red veggies are full of essential vitamins and minerals too.

- *Strawberries, blueberries and acai berries:* These fruits contain antioxidants that help boost cognition, coordination and memory. Acai berries are actually the best choice, if you can find them. These amazing little berries contain omega-3s, are high in protein and are higher in Oxygen Radical Absorbance Capacity (ORAC) antioxidant levels than any other berry, including blueberries.

- *Nuts:* These are another wonderful brain-friendly food. Nuts are a great mix of fiber, protein and 'good' fats that help to stabilize blood sugar levels as well as vitamins and minerals (B, E, magnesium and more).
  Tip: If you have nut allergies, as we do in our house, a great alternative to nuts are Peabutter (a spread made from peas). There is also Soybutter made from soy beans) or quinoa.

A lot of these foods can also have strange textures or smells that can turn your already sensitive child right off of trying them. But if you experiment with different cooking methods (e.g.: steaming, boiling, baking or frying) and temperatures (e.g.: serving a veggie or fruit frozen, fresh or warmed) it can make a huge difference. All of these things work together to give our child information about his food. If his mouth doesn't like things that are cold, his brain will say, "Yuck!" but serving the same food steamy warm with some sort of healthy dip might make all the difference.

How Can I Get My Child to Eat?

I've discussed possible reasons that your child avoids certain foods and what important foods you need to include in her diet. Here are some tips and suggestions for how to get her eating and make mealtimes less stressful for the entire family. Research has shown that it can take presenting a food 30 times just to get a child interested in it. And it can take many more times after that just for her to feel like trying it. That's a lot of times and a lot of meals.

As with anything you're trying to teach your child, the key is to take baby steps and allow him to work through the experiences with the food at his own pace and comfort level. Keep trying and always put the same things on your sensational child's plate as what's on your own, alongside one of his favorite staples or two. That way, hopefully, somewhere along those 30-plus times you're serving that food, he'll eventually give it a try.

The following list is comprised of tools I've used and am currently using in my house, as well as other helpful suggestions from nutritionists and OTs:

- *Eliminate anything artificial and replace it with the good stuff:* This is the number one thing to do before you can start convincing your child to eat what you're serving. Get rid of anything with additives or artificial colors, flavors or dyes and replace them with natural, raw versions of those foods. And don't keep anything they shouldn't have in the cupboards. The best way to get your child to start eating what they're given is to make sure there are no 'bad' alternatives for them to choose instead. This is really difficult initially but things will smooth out and they won't even miss the other stuff (see details on one of the best elimination and replacement food programs, Feingold, later in the chapter).

- *Talk about where food comes from:* As with any child, simply telling your sensitive child to eat something because it's good for her isn't going to fly. Make the foods a little more exciting by talking about where and how they're grown.

- *Show her where food comes from:* Take your child to a farm or farmer's market so she can see where the foods you're trying to get her to eat come from. See if the farmer will answer questions or even let her get in there and plant, weed or harvest.

- *Grow your own garden:* Sometimes planting and growing foods in your own garden can get a child interested in trying something new. This worked for me with things like squash. There's something exciting about planting a seed and watching it grow into something that we can eat.

- *Get your child to help plan meals:* Now, obviously, your child isn't going to choose everything the way you would, but give them a vote. "Should we have peas or carrots with supper?" or "What kind of rice/pasta should we have?" This gives the child a small sense of being in control of what she's eating. A great tool for helping fussy eaters, particularly those living with autism spectrum disorder or SPD, with meal planning is *The Eating Game* invented by Canadian educator, Jean Nicol. Created in conjunction with American and Canadian Food Guides, it helps children put together wonderful, healthy meals and snacks, with mom and dad's help, of course.

The entire system of the Eating Game is made of daily schedules based on age since each age group has different calorie and food intake requirements. There are little tiles of pictures of different kinds of meats, vegetables, fruits, dairy and breads/cereals. There are even tiles for the appropriate number of glasses of water to drink. Each of these foods is color-coded (e.g.: dairy is blue, meat is red, etc.) and there are a specific number of spaces for each food so your child gets exactly the required daily amount of that food (only you would know that part, though). Your child chooses the foods, sticks them to the appropriate colored square on his daily schedule and that's it. Then he can start all over again the next day. This is great for visual cues, motor planning and dyspraxia issues, and also give your child a little power in choosing what he's going to eat. See the link at the end of this chapter to check out Jean's Eating Game. It's a fantastic tool that's helped us with both of our sensory kids' eating issues.

- *Kids in the kitchen:* Kids love to help out so give your child a special job to do, or, better still, see what he can do to help prepare dinner. See the pride in his eyes when everyone says, "You helped make this? Yum!" And this may even encourage him to taste it, since he helped prepare it.

- *Encourage feeling the meal:* As with other new situations, allow your child to feel her food. Tell her to smell, poke, squish or otherwise interact with it. This wouldn't be the best action to take in a restaurant or when you have dinner guests, but at home, let her know it's okay to check her food out if that's what helps her feel better about it.

- *Have a spit bowl:* Again, this may not be an acceptable action around guests or in a restaurant but if you teach the art of discretion at the same time, it can work. A spit bowl is something your child can eject the food into if he finds it unpalatable. The key here is to encourage him to give the food a try with the option of getting rid of it. At first, there will be more spat out than swallowed, but eventually you may notice more and more staying in.

- *Have a one bite rule:* After the spit bowl phase, you can move to a rule where everyone has to try at least one taste of everything on the plate. If it helps, have a food that mom, dad or siblings may struggle with too. That way, your sensitive child sees that other people have texture or taste issues with certain things too but they still have to try them. You can increase the size or number of bites once this is tolerated.

- *Allow him to choose one meal each week that is entirely his:* Again, giving kids the power to choose is an amazing way to help these children. If they know there's a night when they can get exactly what they want (within reason, of course), they are more willing to follow the rules during the rest of the week. My kids loved, and still love, pizza so Fridays became Pizza Night. I used to serve the frozen, store-bought ones or get take out, but after having discussions with Kelly Dorfman, and beginning the Feingold elimination plan, I experimented with different sauces and started making my own crust. Now none of them wants to go back.

Obviously we can't keep our children away from everything out there that we don't want them to eat. They go to birthday parties, their friends have better-looking/tasting foods that they bring for lunch and there are so many fast food and convenience stores out there. All we can do is instill in them an understanding of the benefits of healthy eating, show them the benefits by eating healthfully ourselves and stick to a healthy eating plan at home. Also make sure that you are telling other parents and your child's school that your child has special eating needs so he won't be slipped foods that don't agree with his system.

I'm often asked if it is difficult to not allow my kids to eat the same sweets and treats other children do, and I reply, "Not anymore." With my one daughter's nut allergies, along with my two sensory kids' issues, I have had to be careful about what we all eat. We don't have anything in our house containing peanuts and we make all of our own sweets, pasta, bread, cinnamon buns, granola bars, crackers and other items. It's gotten to the point where our kids actually prefer the things we *make* and, often, they no longer like manufactured products from the store.

So you see? If you stick to it, your child will eventually learn to enjoy the foods you serve. As with everything else, they simply need to learn how.

Different Eating Perspectives, Same Vision

Throughout our journey with my oldest daughter's therapy, I noticed that when we only focused on one aspect of her SPD, such as *only* therapy or *only* OT, we would be successful for a short period of time, only to have her slip back into the state she was even before we'd begun therapy. The key to healthy success is bringing together exercise, therapy, *and* nutrition at the same time. That way, all of your child's needs are addressed in a uniform, holistic way.

I am a firm believer in the nutritional aspect of the sensory diet. In our case, once we removed the unnatural foods from our diets (those with additives) and replaced them with real foods (natural, raw foods), we noticed some significant differences in my daughter's reactions to things as well as her sensitivity levels. Not only that, I also noticed a few important differences in *all* of us. My second oldest daughter, who has asthma and allergies, had more energy and coughed less at night. My son started trying more things on his plate. My own digestive issues (mostly pain after eating and frequent elimination) eased significantly and we all seemed to feel full and satisfied longer.

Many caregivers of children with SPD have noticed a tremendous difference in behavior, sensory sensitivities, coordination and other symptoms simply by modifying the way their child eats. Of course, as with any sort of therapy or treatment, you must try different things until something clicks. And most importantly, you should do your research and talk to the experts before trying *anything* having to do with nutrition and diet. Not only do you want to ensure that your child is getting what his brain needs to function properly, but you also need to make sure that he isn't getting things that aren't necessary, or that are even harmful, to his system. Remember that what works with one child may not work well or at all with another.

There are many avenues you can go down in terms of nutrition plans. I borrowed different elements from three of the best plans out there to help my sensitive children eat better, got the most out of what they ate and made sure that they got real food. Just remember that none of these is considered a diet, at least not in our house. We consider them all lifestyle choices.

Allow me to share them with you:

- *Consulting a Nutritionist/Dietician and/or Health Program Planner:* Though I've already covered the benefits of having a nutritionist in your corner, I cannot stress enough how important this is. A *nutritionist* can help you understand not only what foods are best-suited, she can also teach you how to put certain foods together in the best way so that your child gets the greatest benefits from his meals. In addition, she can teach you about vitamin supplements and enzymes (these help with digestion) if your child isn't taking in enough vitamins and minerals from his food.

- A *dietician* helps with meal plans, teaching you to cook foods in the best ways, and helping you understand what to look for at the grocery store. Dieticians can also teach you how to get the most, and healthiest combination of, calories into your child, even when he's being fussy.

- A *health planner* is someone who can teach you all aspects of good health, not only diet, but also exercise and other healthy living strategies and how to organize it.

- *Following the Feingold Association's Program.* Many years ago, Dr. Ben F. Feingold started his career as a pediatrician, but then shifted his focus to child and adult allergies. He noticed that several of his patients who displayed severe behavioral and/or allergic reactions show tremendous improvement in their symptoms simply by change their diets. Specifically, he noticed that when foods containing artificial colors, dyes, flavors and other additives were removed from these patients' diets, their health improved dramatically. Dr. Feingold then traveled the world to lecture on the importance of removing harmful chemicals and additives from our foods and the Feingold program was born.

- Essentially the plan involves a six-week elimination period during which you stop consuming specific ingredients that are known as high allergy foods. During the elimination period, you are supposed to avoid certain air fresheners, detergents, cleaners and other household items. Once the six-week period is over, the eliminated items are reintroduced one at a time to see if any causes a reaction. From there, you simply stay clear of any foods that have additives, which the Feingold Association has listed in its official handbook. You aren't actually on a diet through Feingold, since you can still eat the way you always have. You are just eating *better* and, as I call it, eating real. It means you eat food in their natural state and only use natural ingredients. Heck, you can even eat candy, chips and baked goods. It's just a matter of reading labels, choosing wisely and cooking well.

- *Following a Gluten/Casein-Free Diet:* This has been a very popular choice for many children who have autism spectrum disorder, ADHD, digestive issues and SPD. Gluten and casein are two proteins that are common allergens and can often trigger sensory, digestive and/or behavioral symptoms. Gluten is the protein that's found in wheat, while casein is the protein found in milk and other dairy products as well as in some baked goods. 'Wheat-free' or 'milk-free' products may still contain gluten and casein, so it's important to read labels, choose items clearly marked 'gluten free/casein free' or simply make meals yourself to ensure this.

The gluten-free/casein free diet is considered another 'elimination diet' because you remove all foods made from or containing these proteins. It can be a tough diet to follow initially because so many of the items we are used to eating contain gluten and/or casein. Luckily, there are now food companies, some of which are listed in this book's Suggested Readings and Resources section, specializing in offering products that are gluten-free/casein free. Many health food stores and, now, major grocery stores also carry these products.

Though your child may understandably resist these dietary changes at first, just remember why you're doing it: to improve your child's brain health and overall functioning and to, hopefully, ease her symptoms. Believe me, it will all be worth it down the road when she feels better and can concentrate more effectively on coping with the sensory issues she's struggling with. And the bonus is that you'll feel better too.

Help for "Leaky Gut"

Many children with SPD and other neurological disorders suffer with varying digestive issues resulting from poor diet and nutrition stemming from restrictive eating. One of these conditions is called, 'leaky gut'.

The lining of our digestive systems acts similar to a colander that filters out large chunks of food, debris and germs while absorbing nutrients and other fuel. When this lining isn't working effectively, the debris, chemicals and other potentially harmful things we eat 'leak' into our systems and can impair our functioning. In children, it can intensify sensory issues, sleep, concentration and learning, as well as interfere with proper development.

According to Kelly Dorfman, healing a leaky gut is a five-step process:

1. **Eliminate allergens.** When we eat foods that our stomachs can't tolerate, they become irritated and inflamed. The most common allergens seem to be casein and gluten. Soy, corn and eggs are also common allergens. Since the stomach isn't going to heal properly while one continues eating foods that irritate it, eliminating the food items that cause the most distress is best to start. That way, your child still gets his optimum nutrient intake because the foods preventing him from absorbing the other stuff won't be interfering with digestion anymore.

2. **Add nutrients for gut lining repair.** Repairing the gut takes a wide variety of specific nutrients to start the healing process. Vitamin A, zinc, essential fats and protein supplements help to encourage the cells in the gut lining to regenerate and repair.

3. **Replace good bacteria.** Dorfman states that good bacteria helps with gut lining repair by helping to change certain fibers in our diet into needed small fatty acids. Health food stores or health food sections of grocery stores carry a wide variety of probiotic rich foods as well as good bacteria, such as *L. acidophilus* and *L. bifidus*.

4. **Kill the bad bacteria.** Once the bad bacteria moves in and gets comfortable, it's difficult to get rid of. A good idea is to talk to your healthcare provider about getting tests on bacteria levels and discuss measures to be taken in conjunction with diet and supplements. Dorfman suggests the following labs:

   - Dr. William Shaw's urinary organic acid test – measures bacterial and fungal by-products. Contact Great Plains Laboratory (1-888-347-2781)

- Comprehensive Digestive Stool Analysis (CDSA) – parasitology test and GI Effects panel. Contact Genova, www.gdx.net (1-800-522-4762)

- Enterolab gluten panel – www.enterolab.com

5. **Improve digestive functioning.** The final step is to give the gut a little help in breaking down food so it doesn't cause any more damage. The best way to do this is to use digestive enzymes. Today there are many varieties, including vegetarian and animal-derived enzymes. As well, it's also highly suggested for children who have neurological and/or developmental issues, such as SPD, to include enzymes that specifically break down gluten and casein.

As Kelly Dorfman says in her article discussing leaky gut issues, "The gut and brain are connected." So if you can help your child's body break down the foods he's eating more effectively and help his gut absorb more of what he's eating, his body and brain will begin to work together more efficiently. And that's an important piece to an overall successful Sensory Diet.

<table>
<tr><td>

8

</td><td>

Helping Your
Sensational Child
Succeed in School

</td></tr>
</table>

Many caregivers of children with sensory issues struggle with the decision of whether to send their child to public school. After all, when your child can't even handle a trip to the grocery store, of course you question how she'd be able to deal with the over-stimulating, often unpredictable environment of the public school system. And most distressing for parents is wondering what kind of support is available for their child in school, or if there is any at all when simply getting the funding for non-school-based therapy and treatment can be a struggle.

When my daughter was very young, her sensitivities were so severe that I wasn't sure whether public school was right for her. I soon realized that children who are that afraid of the outside world would benefit from having the opportunity to practice the skills they are learning. The questions to ask yourself are: Is public school best for my child, and what will she need in the classroom? What should I look for in a 'sensory safe' school? What information do I need to give and to whom? What is an Individualized Education Plan (IEP) or 504 Plan and will I need one? What are my options besides public school?

This chapter arms you with all the information needed to advocate for your child's needs at school. It can be a frustrating road to go down, especially since SPD is one of the invisible disorders educators often miss or misdiagnose. You need to make educators acknowledge SPD and understand it, then work with them in setting your child up for academic success.

Is Public School the Best Choice?

This is a very common question for caregivers of children with SPD and it's not an easy one to answer. It really is a personal choice and depends on several factors.

The top of the list includes:

- *Severity of sensory sensitivities.* If your child's sensitivities don't interfere with his ability to focus, pay attention or work, then he may do okay with a few minor adjustments and/or sensory tools. However, if he has sensitivities on the more severe side, especially in the areas of auditory, visual, vestibular and/or the proprioceptive sense, he may have more issues at school.

- *Anxiety toward social situations.* School is very social and many children with SPD aren't able to handle all of the social aspects of that environment. My daughter worried obsessively about getting too close to other kids/adults, having to speak and otherwise interact with people and even playing with or doing activities with other kids. Her anxiety was so bad that the school support focused on her anxiety more than her SPD. These worries were in addition to her fear of being touched and other sensory issues.

- *Additional issues that affect behavior.* Some children with SPD have other issues that interfere with being successful in social situations, such as social anxiety disorder, speech/language disorders, autism spectrum disorder, or ADHD. These conditions, which also cause your child to have overt reactions to his environment, can cause even greater difficultly for him to learn in the classroom environment.

- *Available support.* This is one of the greatest areas of concern and frustration for many caregivers. If your child has a more severe form of SPD, and it's likely she'll need support in the classroom, make sure that the school has that support in place for you or that it will allow whatever outside therapists you have in place or, at the very least, the sensory tools your child uses at home, in the classroom.

- *Willingness of the school and school administrators to work with parents.* Having the support in place for your child is wonderful, but teachers and school administrators need to work together with parents as a team in order to create the best possible scenario for your child. There has to be a strong home/school connection so both environments feel safe for your child.

It's difficult to gauge how your child will do in public school until he gives it a try. You know your child better than anyone else, so never feel pressured to get him into school simply because of his age or because others say he should be. Compare what he's able to do and what he can handle to what would be expected of him in the classroom, then see what can be done to find a middle ground.

Looking For a Sensory-Safe School

I can't stress enough the importance of parents finding a school that suits their child's needs and not one that the child will 'blend into nicely'. There's a big difference. While federal law mandates free and appropriate education (FAPE), school districts are not required to provide an ideal setting for each student. However, a school that suits your child's needs will be accommodating and accepting of his needs. A school like that helps make changes to the classroom environment *for* the child, not changes *to* the child to fit *into* the environment. That's key to setting your child up for academic success.

When I first started looking for a school for my sensational kids, I thought I'd have to find a special needs school. My daughter's social issues were so intense that I just wasn't sure how she'd handle the social aspects of school. What I soon realized was that although her needs were on the higher side, she needed to be in a place that supported and respected different needs without completely focusing on them. She needed a school in which typical and atypical children learned together, respecting each other's differences and similarities. In her case, she needed to feel that she wasn't the only one and that there were children with different or more significant needs than her own, but also that children without special needs would still accept her the way she was.

For children with sensory sensitivities, school can be a scary place not only because of the different kinds of stimulation that they worry will make them feel bad, but also because it is very different from home, their 'safe place'. Plus, they may be concerned that everything around them will be too distracting for them to settle down and get to work. These include other kids, schedules, hallway bells, brightly colored pictures on the wall, people walking around the classroom or in the hallways, having to sit in a hard chair and so many other things that other people wouldn't even notice.

In addition to all of these things, Carol Stock Kranowitz also points out that children with SPD struggle in school environments because:

- The home and school environments can be very different, with one being 'safe' and predictable while the other triggers anxiety.

- Many teachers or school staff either don't understand SPD or haven't heard of it, so they have no idea how to help your child and offer him the best possible learning environment.

- Even when teachers do know about SPD, they aren't completely versed in what 'good' sensory input is for these children. Plus, since every child with SPD is affected by it a little differently, and they all need different sorts of sensory input to stay regulated, your child's individual needs may be overlooked or they may be getting too much stimulation and experience sensory overload.

- Although many things about school are routine (e.g.: library day, gym, recess, etc.), other sudden changes, such as substitute teacher, fire drills, assemblies or simply having to stop one subject to move right into another can be very hard for children with transitional issues.

- There's a great deal of pressure to 'make good grades' and 'do better' which is extremely stressful for *any* child but especially for one that truly may be doing his best but still isn't 'good enough'.

When researching suitable schools, familiarize yourself with all the people who'll be involved with your child, such as the principal, the main teacher, special educator or related service-provider, and any extracurricular teachers (e.g.: music, art, gym, etc.). Observe them in action with students and each other.

Don't be afraid to ask important questions such as whether they've had special needs children in their school previously and, if so, what options were available to them. Ask if they allow aides such as OTs or teacher's aides to assist your child, if need be. Schools who view inclusion as important are the ones to keep at the top of your list. These are the places that are most likely to be most open-minded to your child's unique needs and to assist in finding what works best *for him* to thrive.

It's unfortunate, but not all schools may be equipped enough, have sufficient funds or have teachers trained to have a child with special needs in one of their classrooms. These are all things to bear in mind and to watch for in your search.

What Information Do I Need to Give, and to Whom?

One of the most important factors in a child's achievement in school is how well the parents communicate with the teachers and other school personnel. Unfortunately, the teachers or the school aren't always willing or able to make changes or adjustments. For example, my oldest daughter was able to concentrate better on a task at hand, especially when it was new, if she could wear a hooded sweatshirt. One teacher actually told me, "No one is allowed to wear hats or hoods, whether special needs or not." I had no problem saying something to the supervisor about this. My daughter used the hood to block out distractions. Once she was permitted to wear her hoodie, she attended more, had fewer outbursts and her classroom work improved.

That's a main key. Parents need to be strong advocates for their child and should never feel intimidated to speak out. As the saying goes, "Pick the important battles to fight, then deal with the rest." In other words, if your extremely tactile-sensitive child is being told she has to stick her hands in pumpkin goo on Halloween, which you know would result in a daylong meltdown, by all means intervene. If, however, your child has a problem with sitting in a different spot one day, just try helping him through it.

Parents and teachers need to work together to help these children find ways to cope in situations where environmental stimuli can be too much for them and to know when the stimuli isn't enough. Most teachers want to do everything in their power to help make the school experience a positive one and they encourage parental support in making this happen.

Here are seven important ways to make that parent-school connection happen:

1. **Arm yourself with resources.** When I first tried enrolling my daughter in kindergarten, the principal told me that she was too old. I'd kept her back a year because I had felt, as did her therapists, that she wouldn't have been able to handle the social aspect of school.

   Contacting your state/provincial or local educational representative is invaluable. Parents should arm themselves with such information as assistance and tools their child needs, as well as any assessments the child needs to have done even before starting school. If parents have all of the reports and necessary documents in hand for their first meeting with school representatives, they'll be miles ahead and cut through a lot of red tape.

2. **Set up a meeting of the minds.** The first step to paving the way for a child's success is meeting with all of the people he or she will be in the most contact with. Once I decided to give public school a try, I decided contacting her potential kindergarten teacher Mrs. P, as she got the kids to call her, was the best course of action. I chatted with her over several months about SPD, how it can affect children's school performance, my daughter's level of it, her strengths and weaknesses and I asked Mrs. P about her personal experience with special needs children which, thankfully, was immense.

   These meetings should eventually include the school principal or vice principal, the child's main teacher(s) and the main contacts at the community funding service who provide teacher assistance, OTs or other helpers or tools the child needs. This 'meeting of the minds' is how the child acquires what he or she needs to thrive.

   Note: If it's decided that your child needs an Individualized Education Plan, or IEP, these meetings also address that. See the next section, "What Is an IEP and 504 Plan and Does My Child Need One?"

3. **Provide a history.** Most schools require a health history. But it's a great idea to also include information on the following:

   (a) *Triggers.* What sensory stimuli in the classroom environment would produce the greatest struggles for your child? Think about lighting, smells, sounds, closeness of other children, etc.

   (b) *Activities.* What sorts of activities would your child struggle with or need tweaking in order for her to participate? For example, think of a child whose tactile sensitivity is so severe that an activity like finger painting would cause a breakdown or, alternatively, a child who needs to feel or smell the paint in order to experience it. Giving the first child a paintbrush and the second child permission to use hands with fun-smelling paints are great options.

(c) *Transition difficulty.* This is a common struggle for children with sensory sensitivity. Be sure to indicate which areas may present a higher degree of difficulty.

(d) *Routines.* Most children with SPD have rigid routines they follow in order to cope with their sensitivities. Discuss how these routines can be incorporated in school to make transitions easier.

(e) *Needs.* These are things your child needs in order to feel more comfortable in the classroom. This includes anything from special seating to calm-down tools to items he or she needs to feel like part of the group.

(f) *The good stuff.* It's crucial to include activities that your child excels in. She needs to be seen as more than a child with difficulties. Plus, the good stuff can be used as an incentive to do the work she needs to do and to remind her of what she *can* do.

4. **Options.** Options are crucial for a child with sensory struggles. There are days when certain stimuli may not affect your child at all while on other days the same stimuli may catapult her through the roof. Teachers need to be understanding with this even when a child is too sensitive one day. For example, for a finger painting activity, he or she can still participate in the same activity but with a few tweaks, such as using a paintbrush or rubber gloves.

   Of course, those of us with children who have SPD and other sensory sensitivities understand that our children need exposure to sensory stimuli or they'll never learn to function in the outside world. Sure, he or she may need to do things in a different way, but the task can, and should, be encouraged.

   For children who are distracted by noise, there is the option of wearing earphones to block out excess noise or seating them away from windows or classroom doors. For children who can't handle certain smells, being seated near the front of the class is a great option. For other children who can't handle being in too close proximity to other children, being seated near the front or on the outside during circle time or craft time can help to keep them focused on the task at hand.

It's all about choosing options that help to *include* rather than *exclude* the child or make him or her feel different.

5. **Balance.** An important point to make here is that children with SPD should never be simply left alone to do only what they find comfortable doing. For the first few weeks of kindergarten, I noticed that neither Mrs. P nor the teacher's aide interacted with her much. They basically left her alone to do her own thing. That didn't help my child as it wasn't teaching her how to cope with the social aspects of school. In fact, the teachers were unintentionally isolating her even further from her classmates. Balance is all about having your child participate in new experiences alongside his peers while respecting his triggers. Understanding the amount of sensory input he needs, or can handle, at a given time is key and caregivers need to help teachers and educators reach this understanding.

   This balance is achieved by making progress in baby steps, limiting the child to small exposures at a time, spending plenty of time preparing for an activity (description and discussion), constant positive feedback and encouraging the child to use his or her words.

6. **Teach the necessity of calm-down time.** At home, we set up a small pup tent for each of our kids where they stored their favorite notebooks, pens, a small light, a few stuffed animals and some books. This is their tiny sanctuary, their place to escape to when their world is a bit too overwhelming. Your child needs a sanctuary place like this in his school environment too.

   At our first school meeting, one of our community funding assistance representatives asked, "Does your daughter need alone space? We can get her one of those eggs from IKEA. When things get too scary, overwhelming or upsetting, we can encourage her to go in there, pull the door down and allow her time to regroup. Then we are encouraging her not to leave the place that's bothering her but instead how to remove herself until she can go back to it with renewed calmness."

   I couldn't believe what a difference it made for my daughter just to know such a tool was available. She didn't use it very often because, for her, losing control was worse than people knowing she had SPD. But she went in the egg several times and her teacher said that by separating herself from stressful situations, even for just a few moments, she was able to regain a bit of courage to try again.

7. **Knowledge, understanding and respect.** These are the most important factors in setting our children with sensory sensitivities up for academic success, each factor leads right to the next. What impressed me the most about Mrs. P was that she believed whole-heartedly in developing and nurturing a child's independence. She did this by educating herself about the child's condition, including the child's form of that condition, then worked with parents in setting goals. These characteristics are so important in teachers who work with our kids.

   This woman had decades of experience with children who have various developmental delays and levels of abilities from basic learning struggles to severe behavioral issues to autism spectrum disorder, ADHD and even fetal alcohol syndrome. She firmly believed that all children have the ability to learn. She explained, "We simply need to discover what works for them...what turns that light on...then bring it out so they can see themselves shine."

   All any of us wants, parents, teachers and assistants, is for these children to thrive right alongside their peers. This can be a reality as long as we give them the tools they need to excel. But in order to do this, teachers need to be taught about SPD and how to help these children in the classrooms, researchers need to further their work in order to provide the data to educators; therapists need to use that data and speak up for children and families struggling with SPD and we parents need to continue to advocate for our children.

What Are IEP and 504 Accommodation Plans and Does My Child Need One?

An Individualized Education Program (or Plan) (IEP) is one of the types of meeting of the minds discussed earlier. If your child qualifies for community assistance or resources of some kind through her school, then the IEP is a legal document used for those resources.

These meetings pretty much include the same people as the other meetings discussed earlier, except that a representative from the facility offering the resources for your child may also be present. The purpose of creating the IEP is to help ensure that the school district provides a free and appropriate education (FAPE) in the least restrictive environment (LRE). There are many levels of restrictive environments, it is not simply a choice between regular and special education classrooms. Consult your local school system officials for specific details.

The IEP has short- and long-term goals created with the cooperation of teachers, parents, therapists and others involved with the child's education. It specifies what your child's strengths and needs are, the severity of those needs and offers recommendations in helping the child reach his academic goals.

Parents should come to these meetings with professional reports and assessment data, any copies of OT notes they may have been given during sessions as well as any recommendations for treatment options. If need be, have your OT or therapist join the meetings to offer professional perspective and appropriate recommendations specific to your child's needs. All IEPs address program modifications and accommodations.

These reports are particularly important because they provide invaluable information about what the child needs in order to function in various social settings in a positive way. Plus, parents are the experts on their child on a personal level so their input in these meetings is very important. Professionals provide the label, the jargon and the tools, while parents provide the loving, calming strategies that work for the child at home, which could possibly be incorporated into the classroom setting.

Here are a few important tips on creating and maintaining a good IEP:

- An IEP's goals should be neither too easy to accomplish nor too difficult to reach. My daughter's kindergarten teacher, bless her heart, didn't want to represent my kid in a bad light so she set easy goals that she achieved, seemingly with ease. If a child's IEP reflects that all goals have been met, special education services may end because it will appear that they are no longer needed. Accordingly, funding can be discontinued, even if your child still needs the support. However, if the goals are too difficult, the child will only end up getting frustrated. IEP meetings can be held whenever it appears that a child's program needs to be revised.

- A goal such as, "By the end of December, Tanya will be able to express how she feels when using the 'How Does Your Engine Run?' game[2] 30 percent of the time, with adult prompting," sets a realistic goal within the child's abilities but still challenges her. (This pie chart is divided into three sections with pictures of Tigger [too fast], Eeyore [too slow] and Pooh [just right])

- Make sure that *all* struggles and strengths are listed, because you don't want anything to be missed and strengths can be used as motivational tools.

- If you don't agree with a particular goal (or something else) on your child's IEP, don't sign it. Parents should never feel pressured to agree to a plan they don't believe will benefit their child. You are your child's strongest ally and advocate. Never be afraid to speak out on your child's needs.

- Don't wait for a meeting notice if you feel your child's IEP needs to be updated or if you have concerns. You are free to request a meeting anytime if you think one is necessary. It is also required that you get progress reports as often as report cards are issued.

If your child doesn't qualify for community support through an IEP, she may be eligible for a 504 Accommodation Plan. The *504* refers to Section 504 of the Rehabilitation Act and the Americans with Disabilities Act[3], which specifies that, "...no one with a disability can be excluded from participating in federally funded programs or activities, including elementary, secondary or post-secondary schooling."

This include anyone with physical impairments, illnesses or injuries, communicable diseases, chronic conditions like asthma, allergies and diabetes as well as learning problems. So a 504, similar to the IEP, outlines the specific tools and accommodations that these students need in order to function in the classroom alongside their peers. One important distinction is that 504s have educational classifications whereas IEPs have diagnoses.

Standards for an IEP are more stringent—including who must attend the meeting and how eligibility is determined. Composition for a 504

---

[2] See www.alertprogram.com for details.
[3] See https://www2.ed.gov/about/offices/list/ocr/504faq.html

meeting just requires somebody who knows the child and another who knows the disability.

A 504 plan removes any barriers to an atypical child's ability to enjoy a regular school experience and allows her to pursue the same opportunities as everyone else. An IEP, by comparison, is more concerned with the actual resources or service the student is provided with. Because only specific disorders or conditions qualify as an educational disability under an IEP, those children who still require assistance could possibly be candidates for a 504 plan. Many children with SPD don't qualify for services or support because they don't have a diagnosis as defined in the *Diagnostic and Statistical Manual of Mental Disorders* (DSM–5). The IEP and 504 plans give caregivers another option.

Home schooling, or tutoring, coupled with strong extracurricular activities are other options for parents who are frustrated with trying to find a middle ground in public school for their children. Both are great options since the child will be in an environment they are familiar with, feel safe in and be able to concentrate in.

My children have been fortunate enough to have a strong support network around them in school which allowed them to mingle and learn alongside other children with no fear. Successes like this happen when parents care enough to educate others in how to interact with their children and when teachers want to learn how to help. Knowledge spawns understanding and that is the most powerful tool we can give people who want to help our children.

Tips for Teachers

The following are a few suggestions for teachers to help SPD children in their classrooms. You can get more information in *Sensory Integration: Answers for Teachers*, by Gina Geppert Coleman, Zoe Mailloux and Susanne Smith Roley.

- **For children who find sitting still for lessons difficult.** Give the child additional ways to move by giving them jobs like passing out materials or taking messages to the office. Do some in-class 'wiggly time' activities like songs with movement, walking around the classroom or hallway. Allow textured seat cushions or yoga balls to sit on, but not for all day as these can interfere with posture.

- **For students who have difficulty paying attention.** Seat students in areas with the fewest visual distractions (e.g.: near the front, away from windows, away from where students tend to group, etc.). Give them a tactile item to squeeze such as a frustration ball or foam ball or have them do jobs that require them to push, pull or lift heavy objects, which helps organize some children enough to focus on work. Recess is important for these children and often it's not long enough. See if there are other short outside or gym activities they can do to release some extra energy.

- **For students who have problems learning the motor skills for writing and other activities.** Create clear but short instructions, praise each baby step, use movement to help explain the tasks, use activities and tools that offer additional feedback when performing a skill (such as writing in/cutting through clay or wearing light wrist weights while writing), give them extra time to practice and learn, send fun-time activities that require the child to use a particular skill home for parents to do with them.

- **For students with sound, texture, odor, light and other sensitivities.** Have a general discussion with the entire class about how some people are more sensitive to certain sensations than others, help the child learn where the irritating stimulus may be coming from so he knows what it is next time, prepare the child in advance for certain activities that may be too sensory stimulating for her, help the child learn strategies during certain tasks or activities (e.g.: using words to say something doesn't feel right, standing an arm's length away from other children to avoid uncomfortable feelings, etc.), and remember that firm touch is usually better for children with sensory sensitivities than a light touch.

9

Helping Siblings, Other Family Members and Friends

As mentioned throughout this book, one of the most important contributors to a child's success is for his caregiver to become as educated as possible about SPD. Once I became as informed as I could about my children's sensory issues and what they each needed in order to cope with their hurdles, I finally felt comfortable enough to advocate for them at home, in school and in our community. And with the right tools in hand, I was finally able to start educating others about SPD, or at least my children's version of it. After all, if my kids were going to intensive therapy to learn how to cope with their sensory issues and interact effectively with their environment and the people in it, then those people needed to understand my children too.

That's what this final chapter is all about: educating parents not only about SPD itself, but also about how they can educate others in becoming supportive of our children. Parents have many questions about getting others to join them on their SPD journey such as: How can we teach siblings to understand their sister's needs? How can we help siblings not feel upset, hurt, embarrassed or angry by their brother's reactions to situations? In what ways can we deal with jealousy over the extra attention the SPD child needs? How can we educate extended family members about our child's needs? What tools can we give siblings and family members so they can be an active part of the SPD support team? Is there a gentle, non-threatening way to help our sensational child's friends understand his needs? How can we prepare our child to be an active participant in his community and prepare those in the community to interact effectively with him?

I answer these questions and more and I offer some tips, insights and strategies on subjects such as discipline, eating and teaching your child how to take responsibility for himself.

My Sibling, My Friend

Before my daughter began therapy, one of the most difficult things to witness was how her reactions, obsessive need for 'sameness' and other battles affected her siblings. They grew fearful of her because none of them knew from one moment to the next how she'd react to them. My son's personality is very similar to his older sister's, the difference being that my son was mostly a 'seeker' where as my daughter was almost exclusively an 'avoider' and he copied many of her outbursts. My youngest, like most babies, was touchy-feely, curious, noisy, drooly and, at times, stinky. For a child with severe sensory issues, such things could be unbearable for her. And since younger siblings just want to be where their older sister is and do whatever she's doing, the sensory triggers are endless.

I questioned for the longest time whether I'd even have more children after my first daughter, not because I didn't want more but rather because I wasn't sure I'd be able to handle another child with such high sensory needs. In the end, I realized that having a sibling could be a glorious thing for my daughter because she needed a friend... a companion... that one person who understood and loved her no matter what her reactions to the world around her were. But it wasn't easy.

I've always believed in the power of siblings and have always done everything in my power to get each of them to bond with the other. My oldest loves her sisters and brother, and was curious about them when we first brought each of them home, but she couldn't tolerate the crying, the smell of the baby formula, having their baby toys laying around (that meant things were 'out of place') or just about anything that interfered with the way she liked things to be.

The most heartbreaking part was that whenever she had a meltdown, her siblings cowered and cried. It's a difficult thing to understand when someone you care about so much wants you around one moment, when the next they yell at you to go away. It could take hours, sometimes days, for her to come down from an outburst like that and her poor siblings, who just adored her and wanted to play, walked on eggshells until their big sister was 'back to normal'.

The only way to ease a sibling's fear or confusion is to teach them how to live, love and play with their sensory-challenged sibling in ways that are most comfortable for her. I call it, 'Planting the Friendship Seed'.

Establish Building Blocks

As Maya Angelou, author of many inspirational books and Oprah's spiritual mentor, says, "I don't believe an accident of birth makes people sisters or brothers. It makes them siblings, gives them mutuality of parentage. Sisterhood and brotherhood is a condition people have to work at." And this is true whether you have a child with special needs or not.

Children have a natural affection for babies. Even my oldest daughter got so excited when a baby was near, she just had to go and investigate. That natural affection is the first stepping-stone that you can build on.

Those of us with more than one child know that including the older sibling in the flurry of baby excitement eases their anxiety. Encourage your child to understand her important role with the new baby, for example, by saying, "You'll be such a great big sister," or "You have so much you can teach the new baby." You could pick a responsibility: "How about I put you in charge of picking out the baby's clothes each day?" Such verbal reassurance can help the other sibling feel he is a part of the whole process.

Our daughter chose the outfits each of her siblings wore home from the hospital in and we encouraged her to talk to them while each of them were in my "tummy" and even let her choose little things for their cribs.

These are the seeds we can plant for budding sibling bonds.

Encourage Play During the 'Quiet Times'

Near the end of my second pregnancy with Jordy, my oldest child still hadn't spoken. She communicated with gestures or noises. The first time she came to visit me in the hospital, she climbed up on my bed, leaned into Jordy's crib and whispered, "Hi, baby." Right there, I knew in my heart they'd end up being close. I also knew that my oldest needed a way to feel she could be around her sister without fear of her being triggered into sensory overload.

Jordy rarely cried, which was a bonus. But when she did my oldest would cover her ears and scream. She also couldn't deal with Jordy touching her, unless she initiated it, and couldn't deal with the baby smells. It wasn't just dirty diapers (which would turn any one off), it was the smell of the formula, the drool-laced pacifier or even her own natural baby smell.

One morning after giving Jordy a bath and she was all clean, dry and baby-powder fresh, I laid her down on a blanket and encouraged her older sister to lie beside her. She was apprehensive at first but after a while she slowly ventured over to lie down. Pretty soon she felt brave enough to touch and hold Jordy's tiny hands, play with her feet and even rolled around with her. And it was my oldest who got Jordy to release her first giggles.

Encouraging siblings to be around one another in the quiet times, just enjoying each other's company, is a wonderful way to develop and nurture the seeded bond.

Helping to Offer Comfort

Once she realized that babies don't always cry, and that they could be pretty wonderful to hang out with when they're calm, I encouraged my sensory-sensitive girl to help me calm the others during their fussy times. What better way to help children with sensory issues practice the calming techniques they're learning than by teaching them to calm others?

Children have a natural instinct to comfort others. Sometimes, if Jordy fussed and my older girl's sensitivities weren't too high, she climbed up beside me and either rubbed Jordy's back or stroked her silky hair while rocking with me. It seemed to take no time at all for them to calm each other down, and my sweet Jordy returned the favor frequently as she got older.

When my oldest became overwhelmed by her environment, Jordy was the only person allowed to get close enough to offer comfort. And most times, she was the only one who was permitted to give hugs too. My heart warms with the memory of Jordy wrapping her tiny arms around her big sister and saying, "I'm here for you. No more crying."

After a few months of therapy under her belt, my sensory girl knew just what to do to make my son, Xander, feel better whenever *he* got upset and what calmed my youngest, Sophie, down. Sensational kids are much more in tune with other people's emotions and feel things so deeply. Some people think that just because many of these children aren't able to handle touch (e.g.: hugs, cuddles, kisses, etc.), that it means they are unfeeling. Nothing is further from the truth. Often they feel so much that it scares them, so they understand how much it can hurt to feel sad or angry.

Children don't need to be prompted to be there for their siblings. They simply need to be encouraged to keep it going. This also helps all children involved to learn empathy for others and to be respectful of other people's feelings. Emotional development is often another hurdle for children with sensory issues so comforting siblings is a great way for them to learn about feelings...that it's okay to feel and express emotions and how they can work through them.

Boundaries

Let's face it. None of us enjoys the touch of sticky, peanut-buttery hands (or drooly hands, for that matter) on our skin. For my oldest, it could be unbearable. The sensation of a light touch, no matter how good the intention, was painful to her. But there were times when she would bump into things or people on purpose or forgot that her proprioceptive system is much different from that of others making her grip, her 'high-fives' or other forms of social interaction so hard that she unintentionally hurt others.

All children need to learn to respect the personal boundaries of others and not be afraid to set and enforce their own boundaries. But sometimes children with sensory processing disorder also need some help to learn how to tell other people that their touch hurts, scares or bothers them and they need to understand that sometimes their own touch hurts others.

Getting your child to be responsible for these actions and to pay attention to how others are affected by what he does is an important skill to teach. For example, if your child becomes over-stimulated while playing with his friends and he accidentally hurts someone, he needs to apologize even if he didn't mean to hurt anyone. If she's spinning in the house to get her vestibular stimulation and knocks something over, she needs to help clean up the mess and, maybe, help you figure out a better plan for getting her that vestibular workout. If his insides feel 'out of sync', causing him to lash out at his siblings and/or friends, hurting their feelings, he needs to acknowledge his actions and apologize.

In our house, my oldest had to ask her siblings or others politely to move over if they sat too close. She was taught to ask her brother not to re-arrange her stuffed animals on her bed and she had to remember that Sophie was just a baby with a smaller voice and a more gentle touch was needed in dealing with her.

On the other hand, Jordy needed to understand that when she spoke in a high-pitched voice, it hurt her older sister's ears. Xander needed to respect that not all of his older sister's things were *his* play things. Even Sophie was taught not to hit, and to share. It was also understood that there were times when the younger siblings weren't always able to keep up with my oldest when she was 'up' (seeking sensory stimulation) and needed to stay on the go.

Children don't always have the social or verbal expertise to express their needs. But we can show them how their actions affect their siblings so they begin to understand what to do, or what *not* to do, the next time. Becoming in tune with other people's reactions to their actions also helps children learn to recognize social cues, which is something my two sensory kids had difficulty with. Practicing these skills with all of my beauties has helped their oldest sister tremendously in her other social situations.

Fighting Fairly

'*Use your voice*'. It's a given that siblings will fight now and again. But the rule in our house has always been to fight fairly. This means no yelling or hitting but listening with your ears open and your mouth closed, which can be challenging for a child with sensory issues whose instinct is to react first.

Parents should intervene when they hear voices rising and assist their children in reaching a suitable agreement. But, eventually, siblings also need to learn to work things out on their own. That means parents must step back once in a while and let their children try to resolve their own disagreements.

My oldest could explode going from serenity to rage within seconds and, once there, she was difficult to bring back down. Usually I started the resolution process with a simple reminder like, "You need to make your voice smaller, hug yourself and explain to your sister what's upsetting you so she understands." If she wasn't too upset, she did her best to verbalize.

'Use your voice' was an expression we used frequently. Reminding children to use their voices calmly and talk things out gets them back to fun times soon enough. Practicing resolution in this way is an invaluable skill they'll take with them in the future heated debates. And for a highly sensitive child, it reminds him that, (a) being calm helps him to be better understood and (b) calm words work better than strong reactions.

Dealing With the 'Green-Eyed Monster'

Jealousy is a natural emotion for most children. Children with SPD often have to watch their siblings and peers do with ease the tasks that they themselves struggle with and this can be upsetting. Reactions to these situations often stem from jealousy, which can progress to resentment or, even worse, self-loathing. Siblings and even peers of the child with sensory difficulties may be jealous of the extra attention, toys and special exercises or events bestowed upon the sensational child.

Here are a few suggestions for curtailing jealousy in its early stages:

- Use the art of distraction for sensational kids with SPD when they get upset about not 'getting it'. Keep a supply of things you know he loves to do and/or does well to try for a while, then go back to the other activity after some calm-down time and self-esteem-building activities. Sometimes getting back to a difficult task with refreshed enthusiasm is all it takes.

- Have special Mommy/Daddy time with each child so feelings of jealousy for extra attention won't fester. Siblings have to understand, for example, that, 'Your sister needs this time for her exercises,' but that you'll play a special game with them later.

- Include siblings in the Sensory Diet whenever possible. I always did our kids' sensory routine in the basement. That way, the other kids could come down and play but they had to allow each of the sensory children to complete their activities without bothering each other. Once Sensory Diet routines were finished, I always had us do other things together like climbing on a climb wall, swinging, playing body bowling (see Chapter Six for proprioceptive exercises) or other games.

- Explain to peers and siblings what the tool, exercise or special attention is for. Sometimes jealousy stems from not understanding or feeling left out. Telling them what's going on and why makes them feel a little more informed and included.

- It's also a great idea to include the other children in sensory exercises as described above because the higher-sensitive child can sometimes feel isolated when she has to do all of these special activities when no one else does. Your child must know that she has to do her exercises to help her insides feel better and by getting others to do them with her, and maybe even getting her to lead the group, she will not only feel better about having to do her exercises, but will also build stronger self-esteem.

The 'Couple' Part of Parenting

The usual ups and downs of parenting can cause stress for anyone. But parenting a child with special needs adds even more concerns with diagnoses, treatments, therapies, special diets, routines and exercises, just to name a few. Sadly, there are many couples who aren't able to endure these extra stresses. The extra time these precious children require can take away from 'couple time', time that is separate from parenting, and this can cause fighting, jealousy and even resentment.

Take the time, even if it's only ten minutes, to sit and remind your-selves about why you got together in the first place. Remember when you were a close, loving duo before the wonderful addition of your sensational children and the only way to continue to be so is to keep grabbing that time alone when you can.

A few years ago, I interviewed a couple's counselor named Gary Direnfeld for an article I wrote for *Unique Magazine* (sadly, no longer in publication but it was an excellent online publication for special needs families).

The suggestions, tips and advice he gave were invaluable and worth mentioning here:

- *Remember how things were.* It isn't that couples forget about their relationship, but rather that the unique challenges they face as special needs parents can interfere with that relation-ship. Couples with special needs children have to remember that the child's needs are generally greater than what can be provided for by one parent alone. Two able parents can offer the best resources for the child. Therefore, it makes sense for parents to invest as much as possible into themselves, both individually and as a couple, because *together* two parents can bring more resources and energy to effectively care for their child.

- *Deal with stress and anxiety together.* Fatigue, worry, the child's need for greater time and attention, the constant need to stay alert in case of an emergency, the inability to escape, lack of respite and burden of responsibility can all interfere with a couple's ability to focus on *each other's* needs, let alone their *individual* needs.

- *Couples need time to chat, relax, laugh and enjoy recrea-tional activities.* It's vital that couples also seek some sort of spiritual counseling to address their issues, maintain their relationship, and hopefully, repair their spiritual upset.

- *Realize and tackle struggles head-on.* Parents, especially mothers, often feel that any time or attention away from caring for their child undermines the child's development, or worse, contributes to the child's worsening symptoms. Guilt is also a common feeling among parents of special-needs children.

- In addition to these feelings, parents of special needs kids may worry that they have somehow contributed to their child's challenges. They might wonder whether they could have done things differently over the course of the pregnancy or delivery. They may look for answers to what caused the issues and whether there is a way to cure their child. They may also wonder if all subsequent children will be affected in the same way. Some may even wonder if God is punishing them for something.

- It may be difficult at times for some couples to feel truly invested in their relationship. But investing in your relationship helps you feel strong enough to tackle meeting your child's needs more positively. Be there for each other, be as understanding and as kind with each other as possible, recognize each other's limitations and see how you can each fill in the other's gaps wherever possible.

Just remember that because of the enormous drain our sensational children can put on us at times, claiming some 'couple time' for your relationship is one of the most important investments you can make for your child.

And, in the end, that's so important for the entire family.

Sensational Lessons for Extended Family

It can be a difficult task making other people, even extended family members, understand your child's needs. You may come up against people who don't, or don't want to, see the issues you describe or who think you are exaggerating things or who may even not believe you. There can be many reasons for this but such reactions most commonly stem from misinformation and misunderstanding. How can people who don't live in your home, who don't witness the really bad stuff on a daily basis, truly understand what your family is going through?

Here are some ways to inform your extended family members about SPD and teach them to interact and play with your child in ways that are fun for everyone:

- *Gently inform.* Books, DVDs and other resources are good places to start, especially for relatives or friends who aren't 'buying into' what you're telling them. At the very least, this gives them a chance to educate themselves about your child's disorder and opens up the opportunity for questions and discussion. Knowledge breeds understanding. Just be sure the resource you recommend to them is trusted and comes highly recommended by professionals in the field. The best thing to do is refer to the list of references on the STAR Website in the Resources section of this book.

- *Keep them posted on progress.* If your extended family lives a distance away, they may feel a little out of the loop and wish they could help more. Giving concerned extended family little updates each week or biweekly helps to ease their worrying. Let them know what your child is doing in therapy or at school, what's working or describe some of the things you're trying. This may help them feel like they're part of everything, even if they can't be right there.

- *Tell them what they can do from a distance.* Is there a special piece of equipment or sensory tool that your child needs or wants? See if Grandma or Grandpa can help you get it for her. Have a relative or friend make something 'sensory friendly' tailored to your child's needs. Have them write your child letters, draw/take pictures or call to offer her long-distance support. These are all wonderful and positive ways friends and family far away can still give a supportive hand.

- *Prepare visitors, but not too much.* Admittedly in the beginning with my oldest, I made the mistake of 'over-preparing' people. I told them what drove her nuts, what set her off and listed every minute thing that *might* have set her off. Now, how was a person supposed to find something to enjoy doing in our house when they were so paranoid that anything they *tried* doing might set my girl into sensory overload? All you can do is explain the basics, give the top list of triggers and tell them what your child may need to do in terms of Sensory

Diet to calm down. Anything more than that may create an aura of discomfort for everyone.

- *Always emphasize the positives.* Don't only tell other people about your child's hurdles, you should also broadcast his successes. That is essential to solidifying his self-esteem. Plus, you want visitors to enjoy all of your child's phenomenal gifts and 'can-do's' too. So be sure to get those out there at the same time.

- *Have a list of things visitors can do with your child.* One of the things I noticed with my oldest kid was that she sought out specific but different activities with her father than she sought from me. She wasn't comfortable with having touchy-feely-huggy sorts of activities with him but she enjoyed the more intense vestibular (spinning, crashing, rough play) and proprioceptive (Chair Tug-of-War) activities. You may want to choose an activity or two from your child's Sensory Diet routine that she may feel comfortable enough doing with a visitor, like Grandma or Uncle Gus. That way, those visitors are still able to engage your child, at her comfort level, and she is still getting the sensory nutrients she needs. The visitor gets to participate first-hand in your child's sensory needs routine and have fun doing it.

As the years have gone by, Grams has figured out her own special ways to bond with my children, even if she isn't always able to hug, kids or cuddle. And she always brings a few crafts with her that are fun, easy enough for all the kids to do at the same time and tap into a specific sensory area (e.g.: making cookies, cut-and-pastes, drawing or writing). So, with no actual special training, Grams has used her own intuitiveness to become a 'sensational' Grandma!

The Sensory-Sensitive Child in the Outside World

The world is an over-stimulating place. It can be bit much for the average nervous system, but for children with SPD it can be a terrifying place without the right coping skills. In earlier chapters, you learned some phenomenal exercises, activities and tools that can help lift your child up, calm her down and/or stimulate her nervous systems in the exact ways she needs. But which of these tools and activities can be used when they're out and about? When do we know the best ones to use? How do we help those in the outside world understand our child and his needs? And, most importantly, how can we teach our child how to advocate for herself?

In this section, you'll find a few tips to help you and your child in the areas of discipline, emotional development, eating and teaching him how to take responsibility for himself and his actions.

In Chapter Eight, I discussed advocating for your child in the school setting. You learned how to help your child feel good about being herself in school by helping both her classmates as well as the school staff be supportive of her needs. People are generally more accepting of things when they understand them. Having the confidence not only to talk about SPD with people and answer questions about it, but also to discuss how SPD affects your child and what others can do to help is beneficial to your child's functioning in the real world. It also helps for him to learn to advocate for himself, which is the ultimate goal of the Sensory Diet.

Give information on a need-to-know or age-appropriate basis. Many of these children start their Diets at a very young age. Obviously telling your toddler, "Okay, Cindy, we're going to exercise your vestibular system now," won't make any sense to her. But it's a good idea to share information on what she's doing and why, at her understanding and age level, as she grows. A two- or three-year-old would understand a statement such as, "Let's do 'Kathy's (or the name of your OT) Games now, Brandon," because that's essentially what you're doing—playing. But as the child gets older, you'll want to give him a bit more information about what's going on so he can learn to identify when he needs that particular exercise and also be able to inform other people when he's asked questions about it. Try incorporating a few of these statements or questions into your Diet practice. As with most other things, it may take several times before he responds or asks his own questions but keep trying:

- "Let's go on your swing. That will help your insides feel better."

- "It's kind of hard to do this right now with all of this extra noise, isn't it? Why don't we put your headphones on so you can just hear me?"

- "You know how you said your tummy felt funny before our obstacle course? How does it feel now?"

- "Hey, I know! Let's try doing your Animal Walks with your vest on. That will help your feet talk to your brain."

- "Look at the time. It's been one whole hour. Let's do a few chair push-ups to wake up your body."

- "Do you know why we do this game/exercise?" (Use the name you give the exercises in the Diet)

When my oldest turned five years old, I started talking to her about SPD. Of course I didn't go into clinical details about the nervous system or use other technical lingo, but I started using the exact words that her OT did two-and-a-half years prior: "Your brain and your body don't always talk to each other. So, we're helping them learn to talk by doing these fun things/games/crafts/etc." It wasn't until she went to Field Day at the end of kindergarten, and attempted an obstacle course that caused her to break down because she couldn't coordinate herself to do all of those actions at once, that she understood that statement.

I went over to comfort her, and she said, "Mama, I just couldn't get my hands and feet to listen to my brain. I knew what I had to do, but they weren't listening." Once she understood *that*, I was able to give her enough information to understand her form of SPD then she could talk about it.

Just like when you're first answering those uncomfortable questions your child may have about sex, you only need to give your child enough information that satisfies his curiosity at that time while leaving the option for him to come back and say, "Okay, I get that but what about _____?"

Always keep in mind that these kids are so smart. They know that something is going on in their bodies but they just don't have the right words to explain it. You know you've done your job right when you overhear your child answering questions on their own, using the information you've given them.

Use the Right Words

Again, your words should be age- and understanding-level appropriate but go ahead and use the right words for their systems, exercises and other important things. You don't necessarily need to use 'auditory' or 'vestibular' for younger children. 'Sense of hearing' or just 'hearing' or 'balance' for vestibular is good enough. As they learn more vocabulary in school, give them the bigger words.

You want your child to go into the world and talk about his SPD with confidence. Giving him the right information starts with the right words to use.

Encourage Her to Answer Questions

When my oldest started school, she had a few curious children come up and ask her why she couldn't do something, why she wore her sunglasses inside or why she still needed to carry a pacifier around with her all the time. (She never sucked on that one but used it to smell when things around her were too stinky.) When children or adults approached her, she hid behind me and tried not to cry while I explained things for her. Soon enough, whenever one of her classmates came up to ask about her tactile seat cushion or why she needed to wear headphones or keep her squeeze ball in her desk, she still looked back at me, but she tried to answer their questions herself. Of course, if she struggled a bit with the wording, I always helped her out.

Letting your child answer questions on his own empowers him to take charge of his needs and gives him the self-esteem to say, "Yeah, I have this thing I have to deal with but it's okay." My girl wouldn't use any of her tools at school or in front of people until she started first grade because she was afraid of being 'different' or that her peers would make fun of her. That does happen, unfortunately, but for the most part she was lucky. Kids were curious but they were also understanding and respectful. They just wanted to know.

Helping Him When People Don't Understand

Unfortunately, there will occasionally be peers and adults who won't understand or even try to. Children with SPD often feel things at a much deeper level than the rest of us do, so negative things people say or do toward them will hurt intensely. You can't really prepare your child ahead of time for this because you can't predict when or if it will happen. But if it does, here are a few suggestions to help your child through it:

- Acknowledge his feelings and get him to talk about them. Sensory-sensitive children have a tendency to hold things in more than the average child, so getting him to release those emotions is an important first step.

- Remind her that not all people are like that. "Your teacher/ coach/friend _____/etc. doesn't say or do things like that, right? Don't worry about what that one person thinks when all these other people really care about you."

- If the bullying/teasing happens at school, inform the teacher or principal. Most schools have adopted strict policies against bullying. Yes, sometimes reporting the incident can make things even worse for a while, but stay on top of it and put out any fires as they flare up. Bullies can only be bullies if they're *allowed* to be.

- Teach your child how to take the power back from the teaser/bully. There are usually two reasons people tease or bully. (a) because they don't understand something or, (b) because they simply think the victim is weaker than they are. Your child is using the tools she does because it makes her feel better and if she's confident and proud of that, no bully can penetrate that strength. Give her that power by teaching her to say, "That's just your opinion," or "Whatever,' or even to provide information instead of using fighting words. Usually bullies back off if they can't make someone feel bad.

- In kindergarten, my oldest had major social issues. She was terrified to make friends because she didn't know how those people would make her feel. So her teacher 'buddied her up' with a couple of girls who took her under their wings and taught her the wonderful world of friendship. On one of her most sensitive days, a new girl who sat at the desk behind her starting playing with my daughter's hair. Her close friend, Maddie, said, "Hey! Don't touch Jaimie's hair. She's sensitive!" Bless her heart.

- Knowledge is power. As a last resort, if it's an adult doing the bullying, parents can simply give the person information about SPD, the Sensory Diet, the tools/exercises, etc. I always say that ignorance stems from misunderstanding. Help people understand. If they still tease after they have the information, then they're the ones with the problem and that's what we need to help our sensational child understand.

The most important lesson we can give our children is that, yes, the world *can* be a scary place sometimes. But with the right tools, some knowledge and a bit of courage, they can still make their mark in that world and leave their imprint with the people in it.

Tackling the Touchy Subjects

These are some of the most difficult hurdles for any parent, but especially for those who have children with special needs. When a child is highly sensitive, some of the everyday routine tasks we all deal with like sharing, understanding emotions and feelings and controlling our actions in social settings can be much more difficult. Helping your child understand, and relate to, her emotions can be tough. And how do you discipline a child who may not understand that it isn't always appropriate to smear toothpaste on the bathroom sink to 'feel' it?

Let's talk about these concerns in more detail.

Discipline

This is a tough topic for any parents, but here's the important thing to remember. Discipline is *teaching*, not *punishing*. The goal of discipline is to teach children what they're supposed to be doing and the appropriate way to behave by rewarding acceptable behavior. Children don't learn acceptable behavior through spankings, hand-smacking, yelling or other forms of similar punishment. They learn through example, discussion and acceptance of responsibility.

For children with sensory issues, the discipline process may require a lot more patience, time and effort than usual, simply because there are steps involved and it takes them a bit longer to process what you're trying to teach them. Plus, these children often already have low self-esteem and self-concept, believing that people don't like them because of their reactions. If you yell at them or hit them in an attempt to 'teach them a lesson,' one of two things happen: (a) their self-esteem drops even more, or (b) they don't understand the connection between the act and the punishment. You're dealing with a child who feels things much differently than the average child. An over-sensitive child will be twice as upset as when you began and an under-sensitive child may not even register a spanking or hand smack as 'pain' so the punishment aspect is lost.

The best way to discipline children who have sensory issues is to provide a clear picture of what is and what isn't acceptable behavior. For example, hitting the Bobo doll to release some pent-up stress or jumping on the trampoline is acceptable. Hitting a sibling or parent or having a tantrum is not.

The three steps to discipline, courtesy of our play therapist, are as follows:

1. **State what the unacceptable behavior is.** "It's okay to be angry if that's how you feel, but it isn't okay to yell that way."

2. **State what the acceptable behavior is supposed to be.** "Please use a smaller voice to talk to me and I'll be happy to listen."

3. **State the consequences for what the undesirable behavior is and follow through.** "If you choose to keep speaking to me in that voice, you choose to go to your room for five minutes."

Never give a time-out that's any longer in minutes than the child's age in years, unless you keep going in to see if she's calm enough to talk and listen. Leaving her alone too long in calm-down time without interaction could result in the child losing touch with the reason for it. And try using a different place for a time-out than where your child goes for calm-down time. The former should be used for discipline while the latter is strictly for calming. Your child needs a separate place for each.

What you're doing here is telling your child that you understand that he's upset and that you want to help him through it but there's an appropriate way to deal with it. If he isn't able to follow that pattern, then he needs a bit of calm-down time. If a punishment must be administered, it's better to remove the child from the situation and give him a safe, quiet place for a time-out than to keep on trying.

When my daughter used to be so far gone that she flipped out and didn't hear anyone anymore, I put her in her 'safe place' (e.g.: swing or wrapped up in her weighted blanket) for a specified time or until she could talk without yelling. Go back every five minutes to see if your child has calmed down enough to talk. If she hasn't, try another five minutes. If she has, then go in and try chatting while doing some sort of calming exercise, such as deep pressure massage, giving her a favorite squeeze toy or trying some other strategy that works for her.

The point is to teach responsibility for actions without being hurtful or demanding. It's so easy to lose control, but it takes strength to calm down first *then* react. Mean what you say, follow through with it and pick your battles. And, most importantly, always remember to teach that it's the *behavior* that's unacceptable, not *the child*.

Eating and Eliminating

These are among the top concerns and complaints of parents of children with sensory issues. My daughter was willing to try new foods when she was very young once in a while but somewhere down the line she became so sensitive that she turned away anything with undesirable textures, funny smells or that looked bad to her in some way. Dinnertime became a battleground and usually ended up with her breaking down or throwing up right at the table. I covered several strategies for eating in Chapter Seven.

Here are a few of those strategies and a few more to try to, at the very least, get your child to give what you serve her a chance:

- **One bite rule.** This may not work on very young children, but after the age of two, you can give it a try. Essentially, you serve her something she loves, favorite fruit, yogurt, cereal, plain pasta or whatever most desired healthy food she eats, with something new and tell her that she has to at least try it. In the beginning, even a lick counts.

- **Help make it.** Sometimes it may help things along if the child can help prepare a new dish because then she can see what's in it and experience it while it's being made.

- **Have a 'spit plate', bowl or tray.** Simply provide your child with a designated place where he can spit out the food if he finds the sensation, taste or texture to be too much for his palate. Be advised that this could be a difficult habit to break once started. However, this strategy has worked for some parents. You may want to try it and if you see that your child is making it a habit, you can stop and try something else.

- **Share your own stories.** We all have that one food that is so gross to us it makes us almost gag just thinking about it. Share your own experience about how you tried something and eventually liked it (or at least learned to tolerate it). If he knows that you've gone through it too, it could inspire him to at least give it a try.

- **Expand on what's staying down.** Once your child's palate becomes more tolerable, offer variations. For example, if she only likes apples, introduce her to applesauce, dried apples and other textures of that fruit. Then try the same thing with pears, strawberries and other foods.

- **Try a new food when the child is enjoying herself.** At a park, for example, so she associates it with a pleasant experience.

It's important that children get those vitamins, minerals and good brain fats. Children with SPD are often at risk of being deficient in these nutrients based on their tactile, olfactory, gustatory and even proprioceptive systems (e.g.: if the muscles aren't working well, then chewing, swallowing or even feeding herself will be a challenge). So parents often have to find sneaky ways of getting those nutrients into their fussy eater. See Appendix I for more details of how important this is and suggestions, such as gluten-free/casein-free or the Feingold eating lifestyles.

Eliminating is a really challenging issue because the sensation of going to the bathroom is very uncomfortable, as is cleaning up afterward. Children with sensory issues sometimes avoid using the toilet to the extreme and actually hold it until it becomes painful. My oldest would hold her poop for days. I had to actually threaten a suppository and even follow through with that threat because she would hold it for so long that it was unhealthy. I don't recommend this route unless it becomes extreme because it becomes a cycle: They fear the sensation of elimination so they avoid it. Then they're forced to eliminate and the entire experience of that creates fear of eliminating again, and so on.

The best thing to do is to talk it out. A great way to do this is through reading, drawing and discussion. A fantastic book to use with this strategy is *Everyone Poops* by Taro Gomi and Amanda Mayer Stinchecum. Also consider *It Hurts When I Poop: A Story for Children who are Scared to Use the Potty* by Howard J. Bennet, M.D. It isn't just a matter of getting a child over the comforts of being in a diaper and not wanting to make the effort of getting to the toilet. It's a matter helping your child realize that the feeling of eliminating is uncomfortable for a little while, but it's much better than the feeling of holding it. If things don't improve, it is wise to consult your pediatrician.

Talking about it and being open is so important. Watch out, however, that your child doesn't go from being obsessed with not going to being obsessed with going. I must have focused too much on 'keeping your underwear dry' with my daughter because she went entirely the other way where she'd actually push on her stomach constantly to make sure she didn't have to go. "I can't feel when I have to go," she'd tell me constantly. That can be just as harmful, if not worse.

The key is to help your child be in tune with her body enough to catch when she has to go but distract her with fun activities when she's obsessing and wanting to try when she just went 10 minutes prior. It takes a lot of time, patience and effort. The Sensory Diet helps because she starts experiencing and accepting sensations she couldn't before. That helps her not to be afraid to tune in to her elimination system and let things happen when they need to.

Handling/Understanding Emotions

Children with sensory struggles are often emotionally underdeveloped. Yes, they feel things either much more or much less intensely than the rest of us do but that doesn't mean they understand those feelings or are comfortable with them. The best approach to helping children with SPD with their emotions is to find a connection between something that happens with their reaction.

The simplest approach is to get your children to talk about it. Kathy suggested that we relate to our daughter's emotions and help her put words to her feelings through verbal role-play. During a time when your child is calmer, such as after your Sensory Diet practices or during a break from reading, sit with him and just bring up his day. Then when he's talking about something that happened that you know was probably a trigger, you can say something to relate to his feelings. "You know, sometimes when people stand too close to me, it makes me nervous. My tummy hurts, I breathe faster and I can feel my heart going fast." Then you describe your way of coping with those feelings and how you calm down.

What you've done is named the emotion, described what the body does when experiencing that emotion then offered a strategy to get through that emotion. This helps to create mind-body connection that these children need. What you could do after that is ask, "What would *you* do?" and he'll, hopefully, list some of his tools or strategies you practice (e.g.: headphones in busy places, squeezing a ball to distract from anxiety, chewing on a chew necklace, etc.)

It's important to note that children's emotions are most intense when they're younger because they don't understand those feelings or what to do with them. That's the same with any child. But it's more common for children with sensory issues to react by melting down or shutting down. We need to help them feel those emotions, recognize what the body does and help replace maladaptive coping strategies with much better ones. Always assure him that feelings are nothing to be scared of or hide from and that he can always come to you if or when he needs to deal with an emotion he doesn't understand.

It's so hard to watch your child experience things that cause anxiety. But you have to remind yourself that the reason she's anxious is because she has always avoided those feelings or emotions before so it's going to be uncomfortable to be exposed to those feelings at first.

Kathy told me once that she pushes kids to the meltdown point because she's experienced and knowledgeable enough to bring them back down. This may sound harsh to some parents, but this is how to get a lot of these very sensitive children to learn how to cope in their worlds. They must experience things that make them uncomfortable or they never learn to deal with them effectively.

As your child gets older, her tolerances will change, some things get better while some problems may become more intense, and so will the strategies she uses to cope with her ever-changing needs. What we do today to prepare her for what's ahead will help carry her through, make her stronger and give her the courage to be all that God wanted her to be.

And she'll thank you for being courageous enough to help her get there.

<table>
<tr><td>

Appendix

I

</td><td>

Interviews with Experts
on Gluten-Free /
Casein-Free Diets

</td></tr>
</table>

As discussed in Chapter Seven, nutrition is an essential component to the success of your child's Sensory Diet. The exercises you're doing with her help make the neural connections in her brain so she begins to understand how her body works as well as how to effectively respond to the sensory stimulation around her. But if she isn't getting the nutrition her brain needs, those connections may not happen as quickly. After all, a machine can't do its job without enough fuel to keep it going. And the same is true for your child's brain and body.

In this appendix, I offer more in-depth information regarding the gluten-free/casein[4]-free diet. Many children with neurological or behavioral disorders such as autism spectrum disorder, SPD or ADHD are vulnerable to digestion and absorption issues. This can prove to be a dangerous problem because the accumulation of toxic metals and chemicals which the digestive system filters out for us before they have a chance to get into the rest of the body, can produce, worsen or trigger sensory, behavioral or emotional symptoms. In fact, those children with more severe digestive issues also have multiple significant nutritional deficiencies and metabolic disturbances.

Does every child with neurological issues need to be on a special diet? Not necessarily. But eating real foods and eliminating heavily processed 'ready-made' or packaged foods that have a lot of additives, flavorings and colors/dyes can truly make a difference in terms of overall brain health. And that is crucial for children already struggling with brain issues.

Dana Laake, author of the amazing cookbook, *The Kid-Friendly ADHD & Autism Cookbook: The Ultimate Guide to the Gluten-Free/Casein-Free Diet*, presents some signs and symptoms to watch out

---

[4] **Casein** is a protein found in milk and other dairy products. A casein allergy occurs when your body mistakenly identifies casein as a threat to your body.

for in children who could most benefit from an elimination diet, such as the Feingold Plan or the gluten-free/casein-free diet.

Laake explains that the symptoms of food sensitivities and food intolerances can be broad and can affect skin, digestion, respiratory, cardiovascular, neurological, psychological and behavioral development.

These symptoms include:

- Fatigue.

- Food cravings.

- Skin reactions, such as eczema, unexplained rashes, allergic shiners or red cheeks and ears.

- Digestion reactions such as stomachaches, gas, loose stools or diarrhea, constipation or alternating diarrhea and constipation.

- Respiratory reactions, such as mucous production, coughing and wheezing.

- Cardiovascular reactions including abnormal pulse, palpitations and elevated blood pressure.

- Neurological reactions like headaches, ringing in the ears, tingling, dizziness and tics.

- Psychological symptoms including depression, mood disorders, anxiety, panic attacks, aggression and sleep disorders.

It's scary to think that the foods we give our child could actually contribute to his sensory sensitivities. This isn't the case for every child with SPD, but it can't hurt to, at the very least, replace the artificial foods and ingredients with the pure, real version of those foods. If this alone doesn't help to ease his symptoms, then you can move forward to further eliminate foods with gluten and/or casein. As with everything else discussed in this book, keep trying different things until you find what works with your child.

Following are excerpts from interviews with two different individuals who are experts on the gluten-free/casein-free diet: Krysten Hager, who has been on the diet for many years due to digestive issues and Dana Laake R.D.H., M.S., L.D.N., who treats children with ADHD and autism spectrum disorder. Hager shares insight on what it's like to live on this diet, while Laake gives us reasons to follow it from the professional standpoint.

Q&A With Krysten Hager

CL: You've been on the GF-CF diet for many years. Can you explain the health issues you had/have that led to your needing to change your diet?

HAGER: I had what my doctor thought were stress-induced stomach issues because I wa interning at a TV station where everyone had some kind of stomach issues. It was a while before the dots got connected and we realized it was more than just stress causing me to be sick.

CL: I've heard of many people who've gone on this diet for the same reasons. Did you change your diet all at once or bits at a time?

HAGER: I started off going completely gluten-free because I knew I wouldn't heal at all until I stopped eating gluten. I only went casein-free a few years ago.

CL: How difficult was it to find foods you could eat? Are such foods readily available in grocery/specialty stores or are there online-stores?

HAGER: I used to eat at fast food places that provided brochures of what was GF but I got sick after eating at one. I wasn't sure why, but I sent back and ordered the exact same thing and watched them make it. It was then that I saw a worker who touched the lettuce also touch another person's burger with a bun on it. So that pretty much ended eating at fast food places for me. Just because what you order is supposed to be GF doesn't mean there isn't cross contamination.

When I lived on an island in Europe, it was difficult to find GF foods and I had to have family members send things to me. However in the States, I was almost always able to find GF items. Even most of the grocery store chains have at least some GF options, often in the health food aisles and the frozen food sections. Safeway, Kroger, Meijer, and Spartan stores carry them as do Whole Foods, Trader Joe's and other health food stores.

I had never stepped foot in a health food store until I had to buy GF food and I was shocked at how much fun they could be! I thought they'd have nothing but wheatgrass juice in the non-GF aisle and that I'd be eating tofu and crackers that tasted like cardboard, but there were brownie mixes, cakes, pizza and the best gluten-free/dairy-free dark chocolate that I had ever eaten. It spoiled me for all chocolate. Who knew health food stores had treats?

CL: That's very valuable advice on how important it is to ask questions, just like with allergies. Now, how has it been cooking GF/CF? Eating out?

HAGER: I don't mind cooking now because I'd rather know what ingredients are going into the food than to be nervous about how it's being prepared. I no longer eat out since I had issues even when ordering off a gluten-free menu. One mainstream restaurant swore up and down that they gave me a gluten-free meal, but I had eaten there the night before (I was on vacation) and knew the chicken wasn't supposed to have coating on it. The waiter took it back. After that, I told his manager how on top of things he was. I always go out of my way to be gracious and praise the wait staff so they're more likely to help the next person who comes in who needs to eat GF. Anyway, my meal came back and that time there was no coating on the chicken and the waiter and manager both admitted it looked completely different. You have to be careful.

Elisabeth Hasselbeck has a book out, *The G-Free Diet: A Gluten-Free Survival Guide*, that stressed the importance of making sure you don't cross-contaminate your kitchen and kitchen utensils. Her book explains the importance of a GF toaster, etc.

CL: Do you have any suggestions on how to get started on the diet? How to help stick to it?

HAGER: My advice would be to completely cut out wheat and gluten since just 'dipping your toes in the pool' isn't going to help much. The biggest challenge with going GF is the texture in breads and cakes, etc. Thankfully, GF food has come a long way since I started eating this way. I once ate a hot dog bun with the texture of Styrofoam! But now the mixes you can buy are so good! I make brownies, cakes and cookies that people don't even realize are GF. My aunt said the GF brownies I made were the best she ever ate.

It might take some testing to see which kinds of breads and pastas your child likes. When I first started, a friend of mine said the white rice pasta was tasteless and she recommended the corn pasta. However, I found brown rice pasta to be delicious (and more nutritious) than even regular gluten pasta. Your child might not be a fan of one type of pasta, but I'd continue to try a few different brands to see what he or she responds to.

There are also mainstream food companies that have some GF food. Several will provide a list of GF foods and if you call you can find out what contains casein.

For me, it's easy to stick to the diet because I know how awful I feel if I go off of it and also the damage it does long-term. I don't think it makes any sense to try to slowly add GF food while still leaving wheat in the child's diet because you won't see if the diet is working unless the child has been GF for a while.

CL: Do you have any advice on how parents can make others understand the importance of helping the child stay on the diet?

HAGER: That's probably the hardest since I still have relatives who point out, "You used to eat that." I found when I first started the diet, a relative of mine would respond to my diet as, "Did a doctor tell you that or did you just read that somewhere?" When I explained that a doctor actually advised me, she still wasn't convinced. Trying to explain these things is time consuming and some people are very set in their ways or don't care enough to listen.

I'd simply say to a grandparent or other person trying to give the child a treat, "He/she can't have that or he/she'll get very sick and it could also have long-term consequences." People don't always understand, and it is hard when the last time they saw you, your child was munching on a donut. And they have no problem reminding you of that! It also helps to have a snack in your purse so when the child can't have the yummy-looking treat the other person is offering, you have a backup treat right there to replace it with.

CL: Do you have any favorite recipes or foods to share?

HAGER: I love Tinkyada pasta. I make a lot with pasta. I also like Enjoy Life products, particularly their Coco Loco Bars, which make a great snack to stick in your purse. Enjoy Life products are free of a lot of allergens.

CL: Do you have any final thoughts, advice or pearls of wisdom?

HAGER: It might take some time to find foods your kids like, but it's worth it. For a long time I never thought I'd taste a normal textured and tasting cookie, then I got a mix and made the best chocolate chip cookies I had ever tasted. GF/CF foods have come a long way since I started out eating spongy hot dog buns and what they were trying to pass off as a brownie/chocolate cake!

One tip I'd give is that if you buy frozen GF bread, only defrost what you're going to use that day. I usually break the loaf up while frozen then put up to four slices in the microwave for a minute or two. That keeps the bread spongy and tasty. If you defrost the whole loaf, in a day it'll get hard and stale. You can bring it back with a little water and heating but it'll be much better if you do a few slices at a time. Also, when making a birthday cake, I don't frost the whole thing unless I know it'll all be eaten that night. Cakes lose moisture fast, so cut pieces, frost them separately, then tightly wrap the cake and put it in the fridge.

The best advice is to call or look at a food manufacture's Website (usually under FAQ or the *Contact Us* section) to determine if something is safe. Sometimes reading labels is not enough. I had a jar of what seemed like perfectly safe peanut butter with just peanuts and oil as ingredients, but I emailed to make sure it was safe and got a response that said it was not GF.

I know snack times at school can be difficult for kids when everyone else gets to have the pre-made snack, but most schools are becoming aware of unique dietary needs and often let a parent of a GF-CF kids leave snacks there in case a treat is brought in. If a kid, like an adult, feels they're being deprived, then the change will be harder, but with all the yummy GF/CF options available, there really is no need to feel deprived.

Q&A With Dana Laake

CL: Children with disorders such as ADHD, autism spectrum disorder, or SPD seem more susceptible than other children to have negative food reactions. Why is this?

LAAKE: All health conditions involve environmental modification of gene expression. It is what we come into the world with, positive and negative, and what happens to us, positive and negative. Environment includes what is consumed (food and water), lifestyle, toxins, stressors, medications, etc.

In the last couple centuries of the two million years of human life on earth, there has been the onslaught of huge amounts of man-made additives and chemicals—none of which existed for our ancestors. Testing has been inadequate. Existing food additives were grandfathered in when the US Food and Drug Administration (FDA) came into existence in 1906. It takes decades to remove harmful additives or toxins from use. Rachel Carson's book *Silent Spring* in the 1960's and animal researchers gave us the warning that the epigenetic changes being seen among animals would impact humans eventually. That day arrived long ago, and most of the medical community is still not aware of the impact.

It is about the 'total load'. Total load involves all of the challenges to a child's system: illnesses, medications, environmental toxins, vaccines, neurotoxin contents and manner of delivery and diet.

Recently the FDA acknowledged that mercury in amalgam fillings is neurotoxic to infants and developing fetuses. The National Academy of Medicine also acknowledges the connection between fluoride exposure and lower IQ levels in children and is concerned about the neurotoxic effects on fetuses and developing children.

The US Environmental Protection Agency (EPA) estimates that there are more than 87,000 chemicals currently in widespread use, 62,000 of which are small enough to pass through cell membranes. Singularly, toxins may be tolerated at a given level, but when combined with even one other toxin they can become exponentially toxic due to synergism.

There are more than 3,000 food additives, some of which are naturally occurring and safe, but many of which have never been thoroughly tested, or tested in combination with other additives and thousands of man-made toxins for synergistic effects.

The underlying issues involve the impact of multiple beneficial versus harmful exposures on systems that have inefficiencies or defects in one or more of the following areas: digestion, absorption, utilization, metabolism, sulfation, methylation, cytochromes, mitochondria and toxic metal metabolism. These defects can be identified through testing, much of which is non-invasive. The most common findings include:

- Inability to rid toxins efficiently (due to problems in Phase I cytochrome P450 functions. Phase II glucuronidation, sulfation functions and metallothionein inefficiencies). In layman's terms, the tests reveal that there are issues ranging from underlying inefficiencies to defects in the function of the 'disposals' that rid the body of toxins. This renders the child more susceptible to exposures that appear not to bother other children. They are the canaries in the coal mine.

- Low zinc due to maldigestion, malabsorption and higher metabolic need. Zinc affects growth, development, immunity, toxic metal metabolism and removal, sensory development and function, appetite and perception of taste, smell, touch, sound, etc. The lack of zinc increases the retention of toxic metals and the exposure to toxic metals depletes zinc.

- Impaired gut flora, the presence of pathogens (dybiosis), poor digestion and impaired absorption.

The food issues result from one or more of the following: maldigestion, inflamed digestive mucosal tissues, impaired absorption, insufficient production of digestive enzymes, gut damage from toxins and medications, poor digestive flora, gut immune deficiency (low secretory IgA) and enhanced intestinal permeability (leaky gut). This results in malfunction of food digestion, impaired nutrient absorption and absorption of larger damaging peptides and molecules (due to 'leaky gut'), which challenge immunity.

Glutens and milk products become difficult to handle. They have embedded in their structures the alignment of amino acids that when partially digested can result in peptides (chains of amino acids) that are opiate-like structures. These can be absorbed through a poorly functioning gut wall ('leaky gut') and pass through the blood-brain barrier to opiate receptors. The effect is drug-like on behavior and function, and there is a craving for the food sources of the opiate-like peptides.

There are other ways in which milk products and gluten can contribute to sensory problems and autism spectrum disorder. They can contribute to excess propionic acid in the intestinal tract—a substance that when present in excessive amounts causes autism-like symptoms in rats.

CL: What are the primary things you suggest to parents interested in altering their child's diet to ease behavior symptoms?

LAAKE: Some children have immediate and dramatic improvement, whereas others have slower, but steady improvement. Start with the supplements as you improve diet quality and start including GF/CF options mixed in with the typical gluten and milk product foods, then gradually reduce the gluten and milk products until they are eliminated. Improved nutritional status helps change the way the brain perceives the taste, look, smell and texture of food.

CL: As you know, children with severe sensory sensitivities (e.g. tactile and/or olfactory defensiveness) can be a big struggle to feed. How do we help these children eat better, or encourage them to eat at all?

LAAKE: With zinc deficiency, food tastes are impaired and children may even perceive foods as foul-smelling and tasting. The taste buds and taste perception center in the brain do not pick up the subtle tastes of vegetables and many other foods. Hence, the refusal to eat vegetables is often the best sign of a low zinc level. When the body responds so negatively to a food, the child remembers this at the very deep level.

We are neurochemically wired to avoid anything that is perceived as foul or harmful. This is the initial basis for the rejection of so many foods. Perception is reality. The need for zinc in these individuals is exponentially high (25 mg to 90 mg as compared to 5 to 10 mg as a typical base). The typical levels do not elicit a change. The dose must override the maldigestion and malabsorption issues, as well as the higher metabolic needs. Specific testing for zinc is utilized to alter dose levels. As the zinc level improves, the abnormal taste perceptions begin to change and the appetite for other foods expands.

If there is not improvement, it is critical to engage in a feeding program for what has become similar to a 'post traumatic stress syndrome'. The child's system has learned to reject most foods due to the previous negative reactions. The therapist must be skilled in deconditioning. Both are important. In the meantime, small amounts of new foods are mixed homogeneously with the acceptable foods as a way of conditioning the body into acceptance. This is called the, 'Trojan Horse Technique'. It is very effective.

CL: Let's talk about the GF/CF diet specifically. How easy is it to move into it? How can we make the transition easiest for our families?

LAAKE: It is ideal for the family to participate so that the child does not feel singled out. Grains, including gluten and milk products, have only been a part of the human diet for 0.005 percent of two million years of human history and 0.05 percent of 200,000 years of modern human history. They are not mandatory human food groups. What is left?

GF/CF Encouraged or Safe Foods

- Proteins: fish, poultry, meat, eggs, beans, nuts, seeds (no animal milk products

- Substitute milks: rice, almond, hemp, coconut and soy, if tolerated.

- Vegetables of all varieties.

- Fruits of all varieties.

- Grains: rice, corn, buckwheat, quinoa, millet and grain substitutes (potato flour, rice flour, almond flour, hemp flour, etc.). No glutens.

The household can serve the GF/CF foods and if family members want them, they can consume them when eating out. (Note: Most family members also experience improvements on the diet.)

CL: What other things in conjunction with the GF/CF diet help in nourishing the hungry brain?

LAAKE: The brain requires excellent nutrition: B vitamins, magnesium, selenium, zinc, omega-3 fatty acids (especially DHA), amino acids, lipoic acid CoEnzyme Q10 and many more. With nutrient malabsorption, many tissues are deprived. We see low tone in muscles, poor vision tracking/function and impaired cognition, focus, attention and language.

CL: So, in addition to watching for the gluten and casein in our foods, we should also be sure that those vitamins, minerals and 'good' fats are include in our diets. Do you have any advice on how we can help others, such as Grandma, who like to spoil with treats understand and respect the importance of these children sticking to their diet?

LAAKE: Highlight parts of my book for grandparents, or other friends/relatives, to read. Show them any test results that demonstrate the presence of opiate-like peptides, specifically from glutens and casein. Allow others to participate in a visit with the physician and/or nutritionist managing the diet changes. Provide recipes that the child likes and ask Grandma to prepare those. Grandparents want the best for their grandchildren. They just need the information.

Good Recipes for a Healthy Brain

This list includes gluten-free/casein-free recipes, ones that are 'Feingold Friendly', and ones that I have used with high success in my own home. All have been kid-tested and kid-approved.

Chynna's Top Three Gluten-Free/Casein-Free Recipe Choices

Many caregivers of children with issues such as autism spectrum disorder, or SPD have found that eliminating gluten and casein from the diet makes a huge difference in symptoms and behavior. Children with intolerances or allergies to these items often display overt reactions because their bodies simply aren't able to properly digest them. We try gluten-free/casein-free recipes a couple of times each week. Here are a few of our favorites.

Chicken Nuggets (free of gluten, milk, corn and nuts)

1 ½ cups GF rice cereal
4 tablespoons tapioca flour
1 cup potato flour
½ cup coconut, shredded
2 tablespoons sea salt
2 chicken breasts, organic (preferably) and de-boned
2 eggs
1 ½ cups rice milk ½ cup oil (sunflower, safflower, soy, almond, avocado) or more as needed

Yield: 12 to 16 nuggets
    Use a rolling pin to crush the cereal in a resalable plastic bag. Mix all dry ingredients with crushed cereal.
Cut the chicken into desired sizes. Wash the pieces and pat dry.
Mix eggs with rice milk, dip the chicken into liquid mixture.
Cook in oil until golden brown.

Pizza with Easy Tomato Sauce

Pizza:

1 ⅓ cups garbanzo bean flour
½ cup brown rice flour
½ cup tapioca starch
1 tablespoon plus 1 teaspoon xanthan gum
1 tablespoon oil
1 ⅓ cups water

- Preheat oven to 425° F
- Blend all ingredients on low speed, then medium-high for two minutes (the dough will be sticky).
- Cover a pizza pan with parchment paper. Roll out dough.
- Bake 20 minutes. Add sauce (recipe below) and desired toppings, then bake for another 20 minutes.

Note: *This recipe can also be used to make pretzels or bread sticks.*

Easy Tomato Sauce

2 6-ounce cans tomato paste
12 ounces water
1 teaspoon salt
1 teaspoon onion powder
1 teaspoon dried basil
1 teaspoon dried oregano
1/8 teaspoon pepper
1/8 teaspoon garlic powder

Mix all ingredients together and simmer for 30 minutes.
Variation: You can add puréed vegetables or meat to increase vitamins and protein.

Potato Pancakes

3 cups mashed potatoes
1 ¼ cups garbanzo bean flour
½ cup brown rice flour
½ cup tapioca starch
½ tablespoon xanthan gum
½ teaspoon baking soda
½ teaspoon salt
3 tablespoons oil

3 tablespoons rice milk

Mix all ingredients well in a large bowl.
Roll out pancakes between two floured pieces of wax paper.
Cook on high heat on a griddle until brown, turning once.

Chynna's Top Three Feingold Recipe Choices

Although we've tried many Feingold recipes, what I've found most helpful about *The Feingold Cookbook for Hyperactive Children* is creating the Feingold-friendly versions of the condiments and packaged items we like to use, such as taco seasoning or seasoning salt. If you read the ingredients on the backs of those items, it may shock you to see the 'extras' that go into them just so they are tastier or last longer.

Here are three of the Feingold recipes we use most often. And, as we've done, you can adjust them to your family's tastes, tolerances and preferences.

Taco Seasoning Mix

2 teaspoons onion flakes (or minced onion)
1 teaspoon salt
½ teaspoon pepper
½ teaspoon corn starch (or potato starch)
½ teaspoon garlic powder
¼ teaspoon ground oregano
1 ½ teaspoons cumin

Mix together.
Note: When making tacos, brown the ground meat, add seasoning mix to taste and ¼ cup of water until the mixture thickens.

Granola Bars

2 cups old-fashioned oats
1 cup flour
¾ cup brown sugar
½ cup wheat germ
¾ teaspoon ground cinnamon
¾ teaspoon salt
1 cup raisins (or other dried fruit)
½ cup vegetable oil
½ cup maple syrup

2 teaspoons vanilla extract
1 large egg

> *Yield: 18 to 24 bars*
> - Preheat oven to 350° F.
> - Grease metal 13 x 9 pan. Line with foil and grease the foil.
> - In a large bowl, mix dry ingredients and fruit until well combined. Stir in the rest of ingredients until blended. With wet hands, spread mixture evenly into prepared pan.
> - Bake 25 to 30 minutes until the edges turn golden. Cool completely on a wire rack.
> - Invert pan, remove foil and cut into pieces.

> **Variations:** I've also used coconut and sunflower seeds in this recipe. If you want to 'brainify' the recipe a bit more, add ¼ cup flaxseed oil and ¼ cup vegetable oil (Flaxseed oil can have a rather overpowering flavor, so I wouldn't recommend using more than ¼ cup unless you really like the taste).

In addition, you can use the Feingold friendly protein powder for your little one, who doesn't eat much meat or dairy.

Gummi Bears Fruit Snack

¼ cup sugar
3 envelopes unflavored gelatin
½ cup of fruit juice of choice

> - Stir all ingredients in a small saucepan. Heat just until the sugar dissolves.
> - Pour into candy molds then refrigerate until firm.
> - Store the candy in resealable bags or containers (mold for chocolate candies work great, or use textured mold pans so you can cut smaller pieces).

> **Note:** We have severe nut and chocolate allergies in our house so, as you can imagine, holidays such as Easter or Valentine's Day can be a real drag. Although we don't have many sweets as a rule, and we don't keep them in the house, we found this recipe was a hit and use it during fun-time holidays in our kids' loot bags.

Feingold suggests using juices with tons of flavor, like lemonade, mango nectar, cranberry, grapefruit, pineapple, watermelon, pomegranate, lemon and/or lime juices. Apple or pear juices seem to be weaker flavors.

Top Four Recipes from Chynna's Kitchen

I have many cookbooks on my pantry shelf. My favorite thing to do is find recipes that sound great, try them then adjust them for what works best for my family. I also challenge myself to create a 'brain-friendly' version of our favorite foods.

Here are the recipes I use most often, from our home to yours. Feel free to 'tweak' them to suit your family tastes.

Chynna's Friday Night Pizza Dough

My kids love pizza. We used to get a frozen pre-made pie from M&M Meat shops but, unfortunately, we had to give it up when we started following Feingold (too many preservatives). It took some time, but I finally found the right flavor mixtures they all like. The dough is actually our version of Jamie Oliver's pizza dough from his, *Jamie At Home* cookbook.

2 ½ cups lukewarm water
4 tablespoons olive oil
1 tablespoon sugar
1 tablespoon sea salt
7 cups all-purpose or bread flour (or 5 cups all-purpose and 2 cups fine semolina flour)
2 teaspoons yeast

Put the ingredients into a bread maker in the exact order listed. Set your bread maker on the 'dough' setting so you can remove and bake yourself.

Once the machine is done mixing, remove the dough and knead it to get all the air out, then put a large bowl or towel over the dough and let it rise for about 20 minutes. (This mixture is enough to make about four to six pizzas or four big calzones. We divide ours into four balls and freeze two for the following week.)

After 20 minutes, stretch and roll the dough out onto your favorite pizza pan or pizza stone and use your favorite toppings. (Remember: Fresh sauce is best!)

Note: If you don't have a bread maker and have the patience to do it the old-fashioned way, measure out your water, then put the salt, sugar, olive oil and yeast into it. Let that mixture sit for a few minutes while you measure out your flour(s), making a little well in the middle. Then pour your liquids in the middle, gradually mixing the flour with the liquid until you have formed a nice ball. Then you would let rise, etc., just as above.

Banana Crackers

2 cups all-purpose flour
¼ teaspoon salt
1/8 teaspoon baking soda
6 tablespoons butter
1 large banana
2 tablespoons honey
2 tablespoons warm water

Combine the flour, salt and baking soda in a large bowl. Cut the butter in until the mixture resembles coarse meal. Add the banana and blend well.

In a separate bowl, dissolve the honey in the warm water. Slowly add the honey mixture to the flour mixture and blend to form dough that holds together in a ball.

Divide the dough into two equal parts and roll the dough thinly. Cut into shapes (we do squares), then arrange the crackers on a lightly greased cookie sheet. Prick each cracker in two or three places with a fork.

Bake for 15 to 20 minutes, flipping them once during baking. They're done when medium brown.

Awesome BBQ Sauce

2 cups 'friendly' ketchup
½ cup water
½ cup apple cider vinegar
¼ cup brown sugar
3 tablespoons yellow mustard
1 tablespoon onion powder
1 tablespoon garlic powder (or 2 minced garlic cloves)
1 teaspoon cayenne

- Combine all ingredients in a saucepan over low heat. Stirring occasionally, allow to simmer for 20 minutes. Sauce should be thin, but not watery.

- Allow to cool. Store in the refrigerator in an airtight container or jar.

- (If you let it sit for a day before eating, it's great!)

Tortilla-Black Bean Bake

This meal is low in fat (if you use reduced-fat cheese) and high in fiber. Try out different beans, tortillas and cheeses to get your kids to gobble them up. This makes enough for a great meal and tons of leftovers and it freezes really well.

2 large onions
1 ½ cups red, green, orange or yellow peppers (or combination), chopped
1 can chopped tomatoes
¾ jar picante sauce
2 teaspoons ground cumin
2 minced garlic cloves
1 16-can rinsed and drained beans (black red or white kidney, lentil or combination)
10x 7-inch tortillas
1 cups shredded cheese (regular or low-fat), such as Monterey Jack, cheddar, mozzarella or combination

- Preheat oven to 350.

- In a large skillet, combine onions, peppers, tomatoes, picante sauce, cumin and garlic. Bring to boil then reduce heat, simmering for 10 minutes. Add beans.

- Grease a 2-quart rectangular baking dish. Start by spreading 1/3 of the mixture onto the bottom, add some of the cheese, then top with three tortillas, overlapping if needed. Add another 1/3 of the mixture, cheese and tortillas. Add rest of mixture and cheese, with a layer of tortillas on top.

- Cover with foil and bake for 35 to 40 minutes.

- When done baking, sprinkle some cheese over the top and let stand for 10 minutes until cool. If desired, add sour cream or Greek plain yogurt and salsa as toppings.

A Sensory Diet Success Story: A Parent's Perspective

The following contribution is from a parent, Jennifer Kaylor, who worked hard with her son to create a Sensory Diet that helped ease his high sensory needs. She's had, as I have had, wonderful success, and her story is inspirational for those on the beginning steps of families on their own 'sensational' journey:

Jennifer's Story

It had been a good morning, a rarity these days, so I savored every single second. By afternoon things were back to our new 'normal'. Our new normal was that my son was in a complete state of agony and myself in a complete state of bewilderment, panic and frustration.

We were visited frequently by child storms in our home. These storms always had a calm period before they hit. I sat on pins and needles awaiting their arrival. Their consistency was something I could always count on, but I could never predict the when and why.

I watched from the window as my seven-year-old son rode his ATV around the property. He was finally enjoying himself. I should have been happy and relaxing in this moment, but I couldn't. I knew it was only a matter of time before the storm hit. It was coming, that was a given, but what would bring it was always a mystery.

And here it was: Helmet came off and got tossed. Joseph entered the front door, sobbing, and making growling noises. This was due to extreme frustration with the way his clothes were fitting. His underwear was too loose. I suggested changing them. Now he was lying on the floor crying and growling because his sandals didn't feel right. He removed them and put them back on several times, crying the whole time, and they still didn't feel right. I suggested socks, but his sandals still didn't feel right, so I suggested his school shoes. At this point, he was in a complete state of meltdown, growling and writhing on the floor. I sent him to his room and told him he is not going back outside.

My heart was pounding, my head was throbbing and I didn't' know how much more of this I could take. I was completely clueless and at a loss as to how to help my child.

Joseph had been doing the one thing he absolutely loved to do. Wild horses could not pull him off that ATV, so whatever was going on in his body was something completely out of his control. But what was it? I would give my right arm to figure it out so that I could finally give my child some relief from the daily agony that he lived with.

I continued to mention to my son's doctor and psychologist that he seemed to be overly sensitive to smells, sounds, clothes, touch, etc. Neither one seemed to be able to give me an explanation as to why, or to give me a solution. I was completely in the dark.

I had to assure Joseph's principal and teacher that it was okay for him to go home on the school bus without wearing his winter coat. Joseph couldn't tolerate the feeling of layered clothing on his skin. It was only a five-minute bus ride, so he would not freeze, and if he did, well, that would be much more comfortable to him that wearing a coat over a long-sleeved shirt, guaranteed. Not to mention that it would save me an entire afternoon of him freaking out over having been forced to wear a coat that made him uncomfortable because of a single wrinkle in the fabric.

In one of my many meetings with our school, I was asked if I would consent to allowing the school's occupational therapist (OT) to test Joseph for sensory sensitivities. The process of finally getting some answers, and help for my son's sensory sensitivities, began on that day. Joseph was found, in the words of the OT, to be severely affected by sensory issues. Joseph's sensory sensitivities not only impacted him adversely at home, but they also greatly interfered with his ability to socialize and learn at school.

So, alas, a new phrase was added to my vocabulary: *Sensory Diet*. These two very important words would change Joseph's quality of life immensely. I learned that a Sensory Diet had nothing to do with food, but instead, had to do with giving Joseph's body the input in needed so that he could stay regulated during the day. I could now begin to predict the when and why of the storms that had been ravaging our home for so long.

Joseph's Sensory Diet included activities designed specifically to help him and his particular areas of struggle. For example, he had severe tactile defensiveness. His skin was so sensitive to touch and clothing textures that it was a nightmare to dress him each morning. Dressing included writhing on the floor screaming and growling because of the way his clothes felt on his skin. He could not stand to be tickled, kissed or hugged. I couldn't hold my son or comfort him because my touch caused him extreme discomfort.

His OT trained me in a brushing protocol. The Wilburger Brushing Protocol is a program that addresses sensory disorganization issues. Each session starts with the use of a special sensory brush that is used to provide moderate pressure along each arm length, the back then each leg. After the brush strokes are completed, the therapist or parent applies a series of joint compressions to the child. It is critical that parents learn this strategy from an OT or other trained professional, otherwise it could cause distress for the child.

It was necessary to follow this particular protocol to the letter. Proper training in the technique and absolute consistency was a must for it to work. This took several weeks of daily brushing followed by deep pressure. The result was life-changing for Joseph. After each session he could better tolerate clothing and unexpected touch. He was much less sensitive, thus resulting in fewer meltdowns. (I need to mention that this part of his Sensory Diet is not right for every child with SPD or tactile defensiveness. Only your OT can determine if it is appropriate to pursue. The same goes for the rest of his Sensory Diet. It is designed specifically for his individual needs. Those needs can change over time, so his Sensory Diet changes with them.)

I get dizzy and sick to my stomach just thinking about spinning. But for Joseph, spinning gave his body several hours of organizing input. It helped him to stay focused and on task. It also helped him to keep his feet on the ground, so to speak. Without it his body was constantly craving and seeking the input it needed to function. This might result in him rocking, tipping or spinning in his chair. His body didn't know that it should wait until recess or after dinner to get this input.

Joseph's body didn't know that it was inappropriate to get input by doing a cannon ball on the nearest chair, child or table. The impact of jumping and banging into things was proprioceptive input to his joints and muscles. When his tank of input was depleted, his body needed it *now*, and his body didn't care how it got it. When he was in this state, his brain seemed to shut off and he had little to no control over his actions, no matter how dangerous. I learned that it is much better to keep his input tank on full rather than wait until it is empty, which results in injuries or a meltdown.

Joseph responds very well to oral input. I was mortified when his teacher informed me that they were giving him gum. My eyes grew wide and all I could picture in my mind was gum in the clothes dryer and all over everything. Gum at school? Gum was strictly banned in school when I was growing up, so this was new. What gum did was provide oral input. This oral input in turn provided organizing input to Joseph's brain. With that organizing input, he was better able to focus and concentrate on his handwriting, a very difficult task for him. We also use carrot sticks, nuts or other crunchy foods to help with concentration when doing schoolwork. Crunchy foods, a chewy stick or a chewy band replaces chewing on his clothing or small toys that don't belong in his mouth.

With the help of Joseph's OT, I now know specifically what his sensory sensitivities are. Knowing his triggers, I can predict what might put him into a state of sensory overload. I can be proactive and provide his body with the necessary input it needs to stay regulated during the day, for the most part that is. Roadblocks and potholes still get in our way from time to time.

Joseph is now at a point where he can recognize when his 'engine' is running too high, just right or too low. (His OT refers to his body as an engine to better help him understand it.) I can now ask him how his engine is running. If it is too high, he can tell me and access the appropriate tool to regulate it. For example, his weighted blanket and a quiet room. If his engine is too low and he needs to wake his body up, he can jump on the trampoline. If his day at school was too overwhelming, he crawls into his body sock. Stretching in his body sock, made of Lycra, provides pressure/input to his muscles and joints and, at the same time, removes all visual stimulation. It's a two for one.

Joseph is no longer in a complete state of agony. Smiles have replaced the tears and a body sock or weighted blanket have replaced the growling and writhing on the floor. A trampoline has replaced cannonballs on the furniture, off the furniture and even through the furniture. A Sensory Diet has changed Joseph's life in ways I could only dream of in the beginning. Joseph gets to jump, spin and squish his body into a state of calm regulation every day.

Who knew a diet could be so much fun!

Jennifer Kaylor
Proud mother of two SPD kiddos

Suggested Reading and References

I referred to a fair amount of books and resources throughout the book that have helped me tremendously, not only in writing this book for parents but also research I conducted on my own children. If you are ever in doubt, confused or not quite sure what to do, grab onto one of these valuable tools.

Read all material that pertains to your child's situation, check out the websites, join groups where you can share your questions, concerns, battles and achievements or try getting into contact with some experts in the field. Inform yourself as best you can because, as I discovered, the more knowledge you have the stronger you can advocate for your child. And, eventually, he or she will be able to advocate for themselves.

Parents of sensory sensitive children are very fortunate in this time as there really wasn't as much information when I started out with my children. The more parents share their experiences and stories, the more support there will be for all of us.

Good luck!

References

(*Feeding Problems and Preschool Intelligence Scores: A Study Using the Co-Twin Method*. Anne M. Brown & Adam P. Matheny, Jr. *American Journal of Clinical Nutrition* 24 Oct. 1971, 1207-09).

Chapter 1

Ayres, A. J., Robbins, J., & McAtee, S. (2018). *Sensory integration and the child: understanding hidden sensory challenges*. Los Angeles, CA: Western Psychological Services. Chapter One, "What is Sensory Integration?" and Chapter Three, "The Nervous System Within: Understanding How the Brain Works and the Importance of Sensation." This is a fantastic resource for parents who want to learn more about the brain and brain functions as well as how SPD interferes with these functions.

Davies, P. L., & Gavin, W. J. (2007). Validating the Diagnosis of Sensory Processing Disorders Using EEG Technology. *American*

Journal of Occupational Therapy, *61*(2), 176–189. doi: 10.5014/ajot.61.2.176

Schaaf, R. C., Miller, L. J., Seawell, D., & Okeefe, S. (2003). Children With Disturbances in Sensory Processing: A Pilot Study Examining the Role of the Parasympathetic Nervous System. *American Journal of Occupational Therapy*, *57*(4), 442–449. doi: 10.5014/ajot.57.4.442

Chapter 2

Koomar, J., Kranowitz, C. S., Szklut, S., et al. (2014). *Answers to questions teachers ask about sensory integration (including sensory processing disorder): Forms, checklists, and practical tools for teachers and parents.* Arlington, TX: Sensory World.

Pinel, J. P. J., & Barnes, S. J. (2018). *Biopsychology.* Pearson. Chapters three and four for information about the visceral system. New York: Pearson.

www.sensorysmart.com – Lindsey Beil and Nancy Peske's website contains OT information, tips on how to advocate for a child at home and at school, checklists and so much more.

www.spdfoundation.net

www.vestibular.org – A fantastic website all about the vestibular system, the various disorders that can affect it and wonderful resources, including exercises to help cope with vestibular difficulties.

Chapter 3

www.kellydorfman.com – For more information about nutrition, diet essentials or how to set up a good nutritional plan.

www.feingold.org – This is an amazing program that teaches people how to get back to basics in terms of eating. Not only do people learn how to cook and eat naturally, but they also learn about the harmful chemicals, dyes, colors and flavorings in our food and how to eliminate such foods from our diets.

www.braingym.org – Works with the same idea as Play Therapy but also helps with learning difficulties and memory.

www.turningonthelight.com/eduk.html – Using ideals from Brain Gym, this Educational Kinesiology site teaches specific movements of the body that can improve mind function. It uses technique such as repatterning (integration of the left and right hemispheres of the brain through specific movements), stress-release techniques and balancing the energy/meridian system of the body.

www.childrensgroup.com – Using the powers of music, like Mozart, to develop brain functioning and to calm.

www.musictherapy.ca – Music has always been one of the most calming things for Jaimie. Music seems to be good for the brain development and auditory integration and it also helps reduce stress and anxiety.

Chapter 4

Angermeier, P., Krzyzanowski, J., Moir, K. K., & Krzyzanowski, C. (1998). *Learning in motion*. Las Vegas, NV: Sensory Resources. – This book was written for the teachers with sensory sensitive children in the classroom but we've used several versions of the suggested activities at home.

Arnwine, B., & McCoy, O. (2007). *Starting sensory integration therapy: Fun activities that won't destroy your home or classroom!*. Arlington, Tex: Future Horizons.

Ganz, J. S. (2013). *Sensory integration strategies for parents: SI at home and school*. Prospect, CT: Biographical Publishing Co. Particularly the chapter on Sensory Integration Activities.

Greenspan, S. I., Wieder, S., & Simons, R. (1998). *The child with special needs: Encouraging intellectual and emotional growth*. *Reading, Mass: Addison-Wesley*. Specifically Chapters Eight through Twelve.

Kaduson, H., & Schaefer, C. (2006). *Short-term play therapy for children, Second Edition*. New York: Guilford Publications.

Kranowitz, C. S. (2011). *The out-of-sync child: Recognizing and coping with sensory processing disorder*. South Burlington, VT: Paw Prints.

Landreth, G. L. (2012). *Play therapy: The art of the relationship*. New York: Routledge.

Schaefer, C. (2013). *Therapeutic powers of play: 20 core agents of change. Northvale,* NJ: Jason Aronson.

Chapter 7

Compart, P. J., & Laake, D. G. (2020). The kid-friendly ADHD & autism cookbook: The ultimate guide to diets that work. http://dhaomega3.org – DHA/EPS Omega-3 Institute

www.feingold.org – *Feingold Family Favorites* is a collection of recipes by the friends and family of the Feingold Association. Also includes information about the program and how to join.

www.healing-arts.org/children/nutritional.htm—Houston Enzymes

www.karlenekarst.com – Karlene Karst is a registered dietician and a leading health specialist. She has phenomenal information on her website as well as links to other resources on nutrition and diet.

www.kellydorfman.com

www.kirkmanlabs.com – Another great website for information on enzymes as well as a store.

www.theeatinggame.ca – This amazing program was created by Canadian educator, Joan Nicol. It's a fun way to teach children with autism spectrum disorder and other disorders what to eat, how to eat and how to have fun with food.

www.vemma.com – This website sells vitamin/mineral packed supplements and multi-vitamins.

Chapter 9

Biel, L., & Peske, N. K. (2005). *Raising a sensory smart child: The definitive handbook for helping your child with sensory integration issues*. New York: Penguin Books.

Kranowitz, C. S. (2011). *The out-of-sync child: Recognizing and coping with sensory processing disorder*. South Burlington, VT: Paw Prints.

Appendix II

Compart, P. J., & Laake, D. G. (2012). *The kid-friendly ADHD & autism cookbook: The ultimate guide to the gluten-free, casein-free diet*. Gloucester, Mass: Fair Winds.

Feingold (2009). *Feingold Family Favorites: A Collection of Recipes by Friends and Family of the Feingold Association*, (www.feingold.org). Kearney, NE :Morris Press Cookbooks.

Oliver, J. (2010). *Jamie at home: Cook your way to the good life*. London: Michael Joseph.

General Resources

www.aapcpublishing.net – Autism Spectrum Publishing Company

www.fhautism.com – Future Horizons

www.chynnalairdauthor.ca – Stories, links to helpful resources, book/product recommendations and a newsletter.

http://www.sensorymom.com – A fantastic blog hosted by Cameron Kleimo, who is a teacher, therapist and parenting coach. There is a wealth of information provided and Cameron also offers one-on-one sessions to parents who need more information.

www.sensoryfun.com – This is Bonnie Arnwine's website that is an extension of her amazing book.

www.sensoryplanet.com – I highly recommend this site for parents who want to be a part of a group of parents going through the same issues raising a child with SPD. There's a blog, articles and tons of information. What I loved most about this site is that you no longer feel isolated or alone in your journey. There are others who understand.

www.sensoryresources.com – Sensory Resources

www.sensorysmarts.com – A way to strengthen sensory smarts. The website is an extension of the book by Lindsey Biel and Nancy Peske, *Raising A Sensory Smart Child*.

www.sensorystreet.com – Another great website offering resources, information and guidance to further assistance.

www.spdstar.org —This is the merger of two organizations, The SPD Foundation and STAR Center, founded by Dr. Lucy Jane Miller.

Books on SPD – for parents

Auer, C. R., & Blumberg, S. L. (2006). *Parenting a child with sensory processing disorder: A family guide to understanding and supporting your sensory-sensitive child.* Oakland, CA: New Harbinger.

Arnwine, B., & McCoy, O. (2007). *Starting sensory integration therapy: Fun activities that won't destroy your home or classroom!.* Arlington, Tex: Future Horizons.

Ayres, A. J., Erwin, P. R., & Mailloux, Z. (2004). *Love, Jean: Inspiration for families living with dysfunction of sensory integration.* Santa Rosa, CA: Crestport Press.

Biel, L., & Peske, N. K. (2018). *Raising a sensory smart child: The definitive handbook for helping your child with sensory processing issues.* New York: Penguin.

Canfield, J. (2012). *Chicken soup for the soul: Children with special needs : stories of love and understanding for those who care for children with disabilities.* Cos Cob, CT: Backlist, LLC,

Dunn, W. (2009). *Living sensationally: Understanding your senses.* London: Jessica Kingsley.

Kerstein, L. H. (2008). *My sensory book: Working together to explore sensory issues and the big feelings they can cause : a workbook for parents, professionals, and children.* Shawnee Mission, Kan: AAPC Publishing.

Koomar, J., Kranowitz, C. S., Szklut, S., et al. (2014). *Answers to questions teachers ask about sensory integration (including sensory processing disorder): Forms, checklists, and practical tools for teachers and parents.* Arlington, TX: Sensory World

Kranowitz, C. S. (2011). *The out-of-sync child: Recognizing and coping with sensory processing disorder.* South Burlington, VT: Paw Prints.

Kranowitz, C. S. (2006). *The out-of-sync child has fun: Activities for kids with sensory processing disorder.* New York, N.Y: Perigee Book.

Laird, C. T. (2010). *Not just spirited: One mother's sensational journey with sensory processing disorder (SPD).* Ann Arbor: Loving Healing Press.

Miller, L. J., Fuller, D. A., & Roetenberg, J. (2014). *Sensational kids: Hope and help for children with sensory processing disorder (SPD).* New York: Perigee.

Mauro, T. (2014). *The everything parent's guide to sensory processing disorder: The information and treatment options you need to help your child with SPD.* Avon, Massachusetts : Adams Media,

Mucklow, N., & Hartwig, T. (2009). *The Sensory Processing Disorder Handbook: A Hands-On Tool To Help Young People Make Sense of Their Senses and Take Charge of Their Sensory Processing* Kingston, Ont: Michael Grass House, 2009]

Books on SPD – for Kids

Kranowitz, C. (2012). *The Goodenoughs Get in Sync: 5 Family Members Overcome their Special Sensory Issues.* Las Vegas: Future Horizons.

Laird, C. T. (2012). *I'm not weird, I have sensory processing disorder (SPD): Alexandra's journey.* Ann Arbor, MI: Loving Healing Press.

Laird, C. T. (2018). *Don't rush me!: For siblings of children with sensory processing disorder (SPD).* Ann Arbor, MI: Loving Healing Press.

Renna, D. M., Stark, R., & Renna, M. (2007). *Meghan's world: The story of one girl's triumph over sensory processing disorder.* Speonk, NY: Indigo Impressions.

Roth-Fisch, M. (2009). *Sensitive Sam: [Sam's sensory adventure has a happy ending!]*. Future Horizons.

Steiner, H., & Fall, B. (2012). *This is Gabriel making sense of school: A book about sensory processing disorder*. Trafford.

Veenendall, J. (2008). *Arnie and his school tools: Simple sensory solutions that build success*. Shawnee Mission, KS: AAPC Publishing.

Veenendall, J. (2009). *Why does Izzy cover her ears?: Dealing with sensory overload*. Shawnee Mission, Kan: AAPC Publishing

Wilson, L. F. (2014). *Squirmy Wormy*. Arlington, Tex: Sensory World..

Books on Anxiety, OCD and Worrying

Bloomquist, M. L. (2005). *Skills training for children with behavior disorders: A parent and therapist guidebook*. New York: Guilford Press.

Buron, K. D., & Myles, B. S. (2013). *When my worries get too big!: A relaxation book for children who live with anxiety*. Shawnee Mission, Kansas: AAPC Publishing.

Fitzgibbons, L., & Pedrick, C. (2003). *Helping your child with OCD: A workbook for parents of children with obsessive-compulsive disorder*. Oakland, CA: New Harbinger Publications.

Huebner, D., & Matthews, B. (2015). *What to do when you worry too much: A child's guide to overcoming anxiety*. Magination Press.

Jaffe, A. V., & Gardner, L. (2006). *My book full of feelings: How to control and react to the size of your emotions*. Shawnee Mission, Kan: AAPC Publishing.

Stallard, P. (2002). *Think good - feel good: Using CBT with children and young people*. Chichester: Wiley.

Zelinger, L. (2014). *Please explain "anxiety" to me!: Simple biology and solutions for children and parents*. Loving Healing Press.

About the Author

CHYNNA LAIRD – is a mother of four, a freelance writer, blogger, editor and award-winning author. Her passion is helping children and families living with Sensory Processing Disorder (SPD), mental and/or emotional struggles and other special needs. She's authored two children's books, two memoirs, a parent-to-parent resource book, a Young Adult novella, a Young Adult paranormal/suspense novel series, two New Adult contemporary novels and an adult suspense/thriller. Website: www.chynnalairdauthor.ca

Index

What would you do if your child suffered with something so severe it affected every aspect of her life?

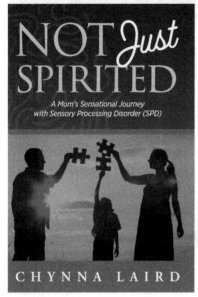

And what if your cries for help fell on deaf ears at every turn? You'd follow your gut and fight until someone listened. And that's what Chynna Laird did. When she was just three months old, Jaimie's reactions to people and situations seemed odd. She refused any form of touch, she gagged at smells, she was klutzy and threw herself around and spent most of her day screaming with her hands over her ears and eyes.

By the time she turned two, Jaimie was so fearful of her world they spent most days inside. What was wrong with Chynna's miracle girl? Why wouldn't anyone help her figure it out? Jaimie wasn't "just spirited" as her physician suggested nor did she lack discipline at home. When Jaimie was diagnosed with Sensory Processing Disorder (SPD) at two-and-a-half, Chynna thought she had "the answer," but that was just the start of a three-year quest for the right treatments to bring the Jaimie she loved so much out for others to see. With the right diagnosis and treatment suited to Jaimie, this family finally felt hope. *Not Just Spirited* is one mother's journey to finding peace for her daughter, Jaimie. As Chynna says often, "Knowledge breeds understanding. And that's so powerful."

"Chynna's memoir is sure to encourage other parents to advocate with the same determination for their own sensational children."

--Carol Kranowitz, author *The Out-of-Sync Child*

"I only wish I had this book earlier. Even though my daughter and I live with this every day, I learned a lot from this book, and will return to my family with renewed hope and energy!"

--Nancy Pfortmiller

ISBN 978-1-61599-158-7

www.LHPress.com

I'm Not Weird, I Have SPD!

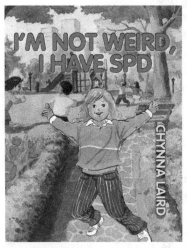

This book was inspired by the author's daughter, Jaimie, who struggles with Sensory Processing Disorder (SPD) every day. It was written to validate Jaimie's feelings and to show her other children feel things the way she does. This book can help children with SPD learn how to explain their disorder to others; help peers understand what children with SPD go through; and also help therapists, teachers and/ or counselors learn how to talk about it. Helping others learn about children with special needs brings understanding to them and help to make them seem less... different.

New 2nd edition includes suggested activities teachers or caregivers can do with children to help develop a deeper understanding of how SPD "feels" plus new pages on vestibular and proprioception systems.

~ ~ ~

"This book is a must-read for any parent who has a child suffering with SPD. It also helps your child put words to what they are feeling on a daily basis. Teachers and other professionals working with children who have SPD also come to a better understanding of how to help these children."

--Tanya Wilson

"When I read Chynna Laird's *I'm Not Weird, I Have SPD*, I almost cried. Not because the story of a child struggling with severe sensory disorder is so sad, but because the frustration shared by child and family alike before diagnosis is so heart-wrenching. Ms. Laird leaves the reader with a moment of with a moment of joy and a real hope for a brighter tomorrow!"

--C. Hall

ISBN 978-1-61599-158-7

www.LHPress.com

A storybook about special needs siblings to engage the whole family!

My daughter, Jordhan, has the unique position of not only being a middle child, but a middle child among siblings with special needs. This story touches on the important contributions Jordhan makes to our family, especially on the days when she doesn't think so. We need more stories for siblings of special needs children. This is my gift to each of them to show how much we appreciate their very important role in the family.

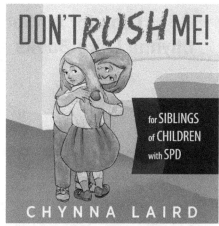

In the book, I have outlined activities that siblings can do on their own, or with parents and/or siblings. To make the most of the message given in the book, as well as from the activities provided, it is my hope that siblings and family members will:

- Have a tool that will help make siblings of special needs children more visible in the family unit;

- Give a voice to siblings that represents how real their feelings and concerns are, even when they aren't always able verbalize those things;

- Help to provide a greater level of understanding by strengthening communication, patience and respect among family members;

- Show that there is so much more than the labels these families are given and offer some insight into how they can learn to advocate for their children; and

- Remember that each of us brings something beautiful and unique with us into the world that we can learn from, and teach others about. And that's so powerful.

ISBN 978-1-61599-264-5

www.LHPress.com

Look for Audiobook Editions of
Chynna Laird Books at Audible and iTunes

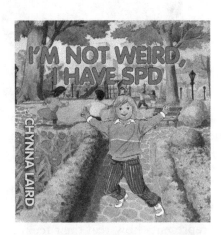
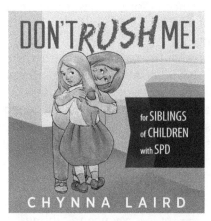
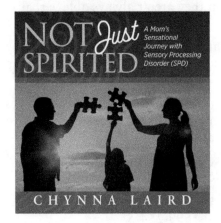
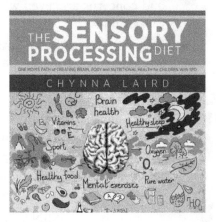

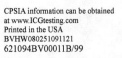